Transition to Nursing

Transition to Nursing

Preparation for Practice

Bill Whitehead and Michelle Brown

Open University Press

Open University Press
McGraw-Hill Education
8th Floor, 338 Euston Road
London
England
NW1 3BH

email: enquiries@openup.co.uk
world wide web: www.openup.co.uk

and Two Penn Plaza, New York, NY 10121-2289, USA

First published 2017

A catalogue record of this book is available from the British Library

ISBN-13: 978-0-335-26382-0
ISBN-10: 0-33-526382-8
eISBN: 978-0-335-26383-7

Library of Congress Cataloging-in-Publication Data
CIP data applied for

Typeset by Transforma Pvt. Ltd., Chennai, India

Printed and bound by CPI Group (UK) Ltd, Croydon, CR0 4YY

Praise for this book

"Packed with practical detail and the supporting evidence, it's obvious the authors are anchored in the reality of today's complex healthcare environments. The journey from student to registered nurse is more like a vertical ladder than a learning curve. This book helps you climb up every rung of the way. This book doesn't just describe the process of transition; it gives advice for both academic and practice based achievement, preparing you to think and practise as a staff nurse. It's a resource you can either dip into as needed, or read from cover to cover. In addition there's an evidence-based preceptorship toolkit for transition which is a useful tool for employers to devise an effective system of support. The experienced nurse would also benefit from this as a reference tool to support their students and preceptees and a reminder of the demands placed on them."

Liz Allibone, Head of Clinical Education and Training,
Royal Brompton and Harefield NHS Foundation Trust,
London, UK, and Chair of UK Clinical Nurse Educator Network

"The transition from student nurse to registered nurse is daunting, to say the least. The realisation of what accountability actually means and the implications of working within the NMC Code (2015) become a reality rather than the focus of an academic essay. This book Transition to Nursing: Preparation for Practice *effectively prepares third-year student nurses for the reality of becoming a Registrant. The book offers useful and practical advice on how to make the most of your final year as a student nurse and how to achieve the highest degree classification possible. The book utilises case studies to encourage self-reflection, and consider how the NMC Code (2015) applies to the daily life of a Registrant. The book acknowledges the reality of working in modern day health care and the challenges that it brings – and offers practical advice on how to develop resilience, mindfulness and self-awareness. This book is a must for all final year students."*

Mike Parker, Senior Lecturer in Emergency and
Unscheduled Care, University of York, UK

"This interesting book takes the pre-registration nursing student on a journey from the beginning of their third year through to registration and working as a newly qualified nurse. The book is divided into three distinct sections, addressing academic aspects, the final clinical placement and lastly registration as a newly qualified nurse. It is written in

an easy to read style using a case study approach with each chapter addressing a specific aspect thus allowing it to be read as a whole or dipped into as the need arises. The areas covered in each section are relevant to all fields of nursing and the case studies are realistic and encompass all aspects of the transition. This will be a very useful resource for third year students embarking on what is undoubtedly a stressful year as they strive to achieve success in their nursing degree and make the transition from student nurse to newly qualified nurse."

Pauline Carson, Lecturer, Children and Young People's Nursing, Queens University Belfast, UK

"Transition to Nursing: Preparation for Practice is an excellent text for all students embarking on the last stages of their journey to become a Registered Nurse. It offers great advice and guidance that will inform and help boost confidence, during the final year of the programme and beyond. The logical structure of the contents and use of case study scenarios allows the reader to develop their understanding of the important aspects of theory and practice requirements at Level 6, and the expectations and reality of life as a Newly Qualified Nurse. This is essential reading for all final year students."

Claire Williams, Senior Lecturer, University of Derby, UK

"Much has been written about transition to practice for newly qualified nurses, Bill and Michelle have done a fantastic job in putting this in one place and producing a valuable resource for student nurses to help them prepare for this part of their journey to registered professional.

They have covered all the important elements of transition including resilience, speaking out, developing confidence and dealing with reality shock culminating in a very handy toolkit that can be used to help manage this exciting and sometimes stressful time !!"

Claire Agnew, Senior Nurse – Clinical Practice Development, University Hospitals of Leicester NHS Trust

Contents

Acknowledgements   xi

Introduction   xii

PART 1

University (or what you need to do well academically at university in your final year)   **1**

1 Introduction to the final year   3

2 Writing at level 6   9

3 Evidence-based practice for the newly qualified nurse   16

4 Leadership and delegation in nursing   23

5 Teaching for the newly qualified nurse   30

6 Passing your assessments   37

PART 2

Practice (or how to perform well and to learn the skills needed as a final year student in practice preparing for transition to registered nurse)   **45**

7 How to prove to your mentor that you are fit to join the register   47

8 Thinking like a staff nurse   54

9 Practising as a staff nurse   60

10 Holistic care of the patient   67

11 Know your speciality   73

12 Leading a team on a hospital ward   79

13 Managing a caseload in the community   86

14 **Effective delegation**   90

15 **Key skills of the staff nurse**   95

16 **Passing your sign-off mentor assessment**   101

17 **Applying for and obtaining your first registered
    nurse position**   105

PART 3

**Registration (or why you should be confident and
resilient as a registered nurse in your first
post as a newly qualified nurse)**   **111**

18 **How to become a valuable part of the team**   113

19 **When to speak out**   118

20 **What the research evidence says about being a newly
    qualified nurse**   124

21 **Dealing with reality shock**   129

22 **Making the most of preceptorship**   134

23 **Why you should be confident**   139

24 **How to be resilient**   144

25 **Toolkit for transition**   149

Index   158

Acknowledgements

Acknowledgements of inspiration to:

My colleague Claire Agnew for your inspiration and supportive advice at the beginning of my interest in the transition from student to qualified nurse.

The research team at Chesterfield Royal Hospital and University of Derby during our years of collaborative research on improving supported preceptorship.

Bill

Acknowledgements of inspiration to:

My colleague and friend, Bill Whitehead, who has not only inspired me but also gave me the opportunity to share my experience in preparing and supporting student nurses in their transition to registration. This is for all the student nurses I have supported in the past and for all those I will support in the future.

Michelle

Introduction

You are at the most exciting, stressful and important stage in your nursing career. The transition from being a senior student to a newly qualified nurse (NQN) is the point where your dream of becoming a nurse is realized and you face the reality shock of finding out what that means. This book is about helping you through the journey from being a student nurse to a registrant. The first stage of this involves proving to the registered nurses (RNs) with the duty to assess you that you are worthy of joining them on the register. The next stage is proving to yourself that they have made the right decision.

The book is divided into three parts, each of which is equally important in achieving the destination of this voyage; that is, becoming a confident, competent nurse. The aims of the three sections can be summarized as the following:

1. Success at university
2. Success in your final placement
3. Success in your first year as an RN.

The book can be read from beginning to end or can be dipped into as and when you need a particular chapter. This book is set in early twenty-first-century UK nursing for those on the cusp of qualifying as a nurse. The requirements of the modern nurse are many, varied and, as a result of scientific, technical and social changes, are constantly evolving. Consequently, the Nursing and Midwifery Council (NMC) identified that this requires degree-level university education as well as many hours of real practice-based experience. Nurse education should therefore be seen as a combination of theory and practice learning, culminating in the transition from student to registered nurse. There is a great deal of overlap between the three arenas described in the paragraph above and learning from each should be transferred to the others. However, the nature of the process means that students will experience nurse education as half of the time in the academy and the other half in the future workplace. In addition, the move from unregistered student to NQN is rarely a seamless and stress-free process as the perception of the individual is radically altered by joining the register. Therefore, the design of the book is in the three sections indicated.

There is a long list of requirements for nursing programmes laid out by the NMC. These include: communication skills, nursing models, anatomy and physiology, psychology, sociology and ethics. However, many of these are dealt with in depth in the earlier parts of the nursing programme and by the third year it is mainly a matter of embedding them through revision and reflection upon them. Some consideration of these areas of essential nursing knowledge and skills will be interspersed throughout the book. Nevertheless, the chapter headings indicate the central issues to be covered in preparation for the student to become an RN. The chapters illustrate these issues with a number of useful features:

- *Examples of good practice* to help students consider how best to deal with situations.
- *Case studies and scenarios* to help students explore key aspects of nursing practice.
- *Reflective exercises* for students to self-test their understanding and application of the material.

We have written this book based on our decades of practical experience as RNs; our years of knowledge as senior university lecturers, teaching and facilitating the journey of hundreds of senior students' transition to become RNs; and our collaborative research involving students, NQNs, clinical nurse educators and preceptors. We believe that the advice in this book will help you to make this big, important step with the confidence and resilience that you will need to become the high quality nurse that you deserve to be.

Gendered writing

Where we have been discussing people in general we have attempted to use the gender neutral plurals such as their, them, theirs. When identifying fictional individuals in case studies we have identified people as male or female in random distribution.

University (or what you need to do well academically at university in your final year)

1 Introduction to the final year

Overview

You are entering the final year of your degree. You will need to meet three expectations from the university: academic standards; professional standards; clinical competency and to achieve the graduate expectations of their university. Assessment of your conduct as well as academic achievement is an important aspect of this.

Introduction

You are now in, or approaching, the final year of your programme of study and may be feeling elated, anxious, tired or a little stressed; indeed, you may be feeling all those things and one may argue that these are perfectly normal emotions as you approach the end of your programme. You may wish to know what your nursing lecturers and mentors will be looking for in your performance and what progress they want to see that you are making. This chapter is divided into three sections – Part 1 considers professionalism, Part 2 considers academic elements of the course and Part 3 considers practice elements. These sections should help you to ascertain what it is you need to demonstrate in this final year.

Lecturers have a responsibility to ensure that the assessments undertaken in the final year of the pre-registration nursing programme test the students' knowledge, understanding and problem solving. The final year student should also demonstrate sound critical thinking skills and that they can utilize appropriate evidence to support their decision making. Their mentors in the clinical placement areas should confirm that the student's practice also meets the competency demands for transfer to the register and that they feel the student is a safe practitioner. At this assessment point, it is vital that you demonstrate your leaderships and delegation abilities. In addition, you should be supervising other members of staff.

Professionalism

The academic and clinical teams also assess the student's professionalism in their approach to the nursing role. Although there is some debate surrounding the concept of what a professional is and the perception that the label of being part of 'a caring profession' lessens that status (Keeling and Templeman, 2013), we continue to demand professional recognition and every nurse has an obligation to carry this responsibility forward into their future career. Professionalism is an evolving concept. Keeling and Templeman (2013) identified in their study when examining student nurses' perceptions of professionalism that while the meaning and concept of what the term embodies may have changed, there are key similarities that have remained consistent. These similarities include the altruistic traits in those desiring to enter the profession, their honesty, and the innate need to care. These are among the key characteristics that the academic staff will look for in student nurses, especially as they prepare to enter the final stages of their programme.

Case study 1.1: Beatrice

Beatrice was in her final theoretical module. She always arrived early for her teaching sessions. She passed her summative viva assessment after doing a great deal of work.

The lecturers noted that, in class, she appeared to be interested and enthusiastic, often asking very insightful questions. She worked well in her groups and often supported members who struggled. Beatrice always engaged in academic supervision for summative work.

Reflection

- How is Beatrice displaying her professionalism?
- Do you think her current attitude and conduct will have an effect on her clinical practice?

It is clear that Beatrice is fully engaged in her theoretical modules and this engagement should have a significant impact on her practice and her confidence. One may assume that she will be attaining a greater knowledge base and understanding surrounding her role and the responsibilities inherent in that role.

She also appears to be very reliable, which is vital from an employability perspective. A manager needs someone who will turn up to work and give the best they can to ensure patients are well cared for and that their colleagues feel supported. Working as part of a team is crucial in healthcare as patients may require a number of professionals to work together cohesively to ensure they receive the required care.

It is also clear from Beatrice's performance in group activities that she has the right skill set, attitudes and values required for effective teamworking. Lecturers will often organize group activities in order to encourage group dynamics, and to manage and resolve conflict within a team if it occurs. These skills are essential during the transition from student to qualified nurse. The lecturer will be looking at the way the group engages with each other and examining the student's ability to work as part of a team. Engaging in this will help the student to understand their role in the group and be cognizant of other members of the group and their roles, which, when delivering patient care, is vital (Webb, 2011).

Professionalism involves displaying a set of positive values. Ritchie (2011) proposes that being trustworthy and working in the best interests of the patient are qualities the general public want of the qualified nurse. Wanting to learn and understand so that one can be safe in practice should be a basic quality that all nursing students possess. To not engage insinuates a complacent attitude to patient care and may even suggest a lack of interest in the well-being of the patients you care for. In this case study, Beatrice has demonstrated that she is trustworthy and wants to ensure she has a good understanding of the theoretical underpinning related to caring for patients. At this stage in Beatrice's programme, she is demonstrating all the key attributes you need to. In the UK, programme leaders (PLs) have to complete a statement for the Nursing and Midwifery Council (NMC) declaring each nurse's good character. Beatrice appears to be portraying all the key behaviours and attitudes the PL needs to declare.

Reflection

- If Beatrice had not yet demonstrated the right behaviours and attitudes, how could she retrieve her module and good character?

If there have been personal issues within Beatrice's life that have had a negative impact on her ability to engage, she would need to discuss these with her tutor in order to gain support but also to clarify her reasons for non-engagement. Lecturers are fully aware that life may be complex and also that the programme for pre-registration is demanding. Rather than present a perception of 'don't care' the reality of 'I am trying but life is difficult' can make a huge difference to how a student can be supported within a programme of study.

Academic demands

Although nursing is associated with skills and practical activity, understanding why you are doing a specific task and being able to examine and appraise the evidence underpinning your care and duties is vital (Nursing and Medical Council (NMC), 2015). The academic content of a graduate nursing programme should fulfil a number of requirements. These include the academic rigour to allow the credits associated with a degree award to be achieved.

Academic writing may present anxieties among many university students. Moving between academic levels again can incite some apprehension among those undertaking academic programmes. Lecturers can support students and inform them of the requirements at a specific level but sitting and writing with those requirements in mind may become daunting.

During the last year of a degree programme, success in producing work at level 6 is required in order to achieve the credits to allow the progression and in this case entry to the register on completion (see Chapter 2 for more guidance surrounding level 6 writing). The lecturer will be encouraging engagement in order to maximize your potential for achieving a high classification. You need to engage in this process and assure yourself that you are addressing the assessment accurately and appropriately. If, for example, it is a literature review and you wish to examine literature surrounding efficacy of leg ulcer treatments, then you need to do a review of the selected literature rather than write an assignment about leg ulcers. Your lecturer should be there to help and so seek clarification when possible. This will not necessarily guarantee your success but it will certainly improve your chances. Academic institutions offer varying support; it is your responsibility to maximize the support available to give you the greatest chance of success. You lecturer will want to see you engaging in your work as you will be demonstrating your commitment to the programme and to your learning.

Case study 1.2: Melissa

Melissa was undertaking her dissertation and she was appraising literature surrounding end-of-life care. She had attended for tutorial support and felt quite clear about what was being asked of her. Her tutor was impressed by her enthusiasm and dedication. She demonstrated a real desire to be a competent practitioner.

When marking her review, the tutor was examining it for a good understanding and knowledge, not only of end-of-life care, but also an understanding of research methodologies and appraisal of the evidence. During the review she applied the research findings to practice and identified how issues may be addressed and potentially resolved through a variation in practice.

By doing this in her work she demonstrated key skills required for progression and transfer to the nursing register. She was able to link theory and practice utilizing current evidence. Kumeran and Carney (2014) identify that competency and being able to link theory and practice are vital in safe and effective nursing practice because a nurse will need to practise utilizing up-to-date reliable and valid evidence (NMC, 2015) in order to ensure that the care she delivers is evidence based. Melissa was also able to demonstrate her critical thinking skills, problem solving and sound knowledge base that are key programme requirements as stated by the NMC (2010); it is worth noting that her university has a responsibility to ensure she is fit for practice in these and other areas.

Practice

As identified earlier, pre-registration nursing is not simply an academic programme but a professional programme that involves a practice element. This practice should not be more important or less important than the academic content. They should be interlinked and reflect the aims and goals in the education of the pre-registration student nurse. Reading Case study 1.3 and answering the Reflection questions will help you to explore this idea further.

> **Case study 1.3: Helen**
>
> Helen has achieved extremely high grades in her academic work. She is on target for a high classification at the end of the programme. During her placements in the second year, a number of mentors had some concerns about her communication skills but found that by the end of the placement she had managed to convince the staff, through her clinical performance, that they were adequate. She was undertaking her management placement and her sign-off mentor had great concerns regarding Helen's communication with patients and team members. She failed to give eye contact and would not speak clearly. Patients found it difficult to understand her and the multidisciplinary team (MT) avoided contact as they found her rude because she appeared disinterested.

Reflection

- What do you feel the issues are?
- What is wrong with Helen's behaviour?
- What does it say in the Code (NMC, 2015) and standards for pre-registration nursing education about communication?

Although Helen was succeeding, even excelling academically in the programme, her clinical skills may threaten her ability to progress and enter the nursing register unless she can improve these, specifically her communication skills. Effective communication between the nurse and patient is vital. It helps to foster the relationship to be able to meet patients' needs (McCabe and Timmins, 2007). Equally, lack of effective communication within a team can have serious consequences for vulnerable patients (House of Commons Health Committee, 2002–3; Francis, 2013).

Your tutor should be contacted if there were any concerns about your performance in practice, but it is worth noting that it is your responsibility to escalate your concerns to your academic tutor about areas where you might be struggling as well as the responsibility of the clinical placement team. Your tutor will be looking for safe practice as well as evidence of understanding and application in your theoretical work. Failure to attain an adequate standard in either of these aspects will affect your programme and the potential for a future career as a registered nurse (RN).

Conclusion

Although the lecturer on your course is not the only person who assesses your suitability to enter the nursing register, they are instrumental in collating the evidence in preparation for this transition. They will be undertaking investigation and observation to answer the question raised for anyone who is completing a pre-registration nursing programme: Is this person fit for purpose and fit for practice at the point of entry to the register? Academic and practice staff have a duty of care to patients to ensure that only safe practitioners enter the register and it is your responsibility to identify deficits in knowledge base and understanding that may have negative consequences for the patients you care for. This self-awareness regarding competency will continue well into your future career but at the point of registration there is an acknowledgement that a fundamental level of skill and understanding is required; for example, to be able to administer medication safely, to be able to assess a patient's nutritional needs, to be able to carry out clinical observations that the newly qualified nurse (NQN) should be competent to carry out. All those involved in your assessment will be looking for these skills among many others and also ensuring that you can achieve the academic standard required for the degree award.

References

Francis, R. (2013) *Report of the Mid Staffordshire NHS Foundation Trust Public Inquiry.* London: Her Majesty's Stationery Office (HMSO).

House of Commons Health Committee (2002–3) *The Victoria Climbié Inquiry Report: Sixth Report of Session 2002–3.* London: Her Majesty's Stationery Office (HMSO).

Keeling, J. and Templeman, J. (2013) An exploratory study: student nurses' perceptions of professionalism, *Nurse Education in Practice*, 13(1): 18–22.

Kumeran, S. and Carney, M. (2014) Role transition from student nurse to staff nurse: facilitating the transition period, *Nurse Education in Practice*, 14(6): 605–611.

McCabe, C. and Timmins, F. (eds) (2007) *Communication Skills for Nursing and Practice.* Basingstoke: Palgrave Macmillan.

Nursing and Midwifery Council (NMC) (2010) *Standards for Pre-registration Nursing Education.* London: NMC.

Nursing and Midwifery Council (NMC) (2015) *The Code.* London: NMC.

Ritchie, D. (2011) Being a professional nurse: image and values in nursing, in Hall, C. and Ritchie, D. (eds) *What is Nursing? Exploring Theory and Practice*, 2nd edn. Exeter: Learning Matters Ltd.

Webb, L. (2011) *Nursing: Communication Skills in Practice.* Oxford: Oxford University Press.

Writing at level 6

Overview

In order to be awarded a degree you will need to indicate that you have achieved academic level 6. This chapter provides practical advice on how you can achieve the required level and how best to provide evidence for this in your writing and other assessments. This is further developed in Chapter 6 by providing helpful support and advice about how to pass your assessments.

Nursing programmes

Being able to write at level 6 in the final year of your programme is crucial in order to demonstrate you have the in-depth knowledge and understanding to enable you to progress and transfer onto the nursing register. It is not simply a case of writing articulately; it is about being able to problem-solve, make suggestions and transfer theoretical knowledge into practice. Your assessments in your final year will allow you to demonstrate this skill.

Historically, the call for nurses to be more knowledgeable and to write using a more academic stance started as a result of concerns regarding the lack of preparedness of student nurses for transition to registration (Maben and Macleod Clark, 1998). In response to these concerns, the United Kingdom Central Council (UKCC) for Nursing Midwifery and Health Visiting (UKCC, 1986) introduced a new curriculum to the UK to try to address the deficits identified that included lack of knowledge and skills on qualification. More theoretical and academic study was seen as the way forward but also an academic qualification (diploma) was awarded on completion as well as entry to the register. This model of education was termed Project 2000 (UKCC, 1986). Although there have been changes to the curriculum and what has been deemed essential in the preparation for practice, greater academic attainment has been key with the phasing out of diploma courses and the introduction of degree and Masters level programmes (Nursing and Midwifery Council (NMC), 2010). Clinical competency is vital as you progress through your final year but also having academic competency to degree level is seen as equally important in order to demonstrate an adequate understanding of key theoretical concepts when practising as a nurse.

The degree programme demands that academic level 6 is attained in order to be awarded a degree. Students are encouraged to achieve high pass marks in their final year to maximize their classification. Although this does not affect your registration, it may have an impact on your future employability or opportunity for further academic study. At this point the last thing you may think of is further study but nursing offers numerous opportunities and sometimes academic study is required in order to demonstrate you have higher levels of expertise, theoretical and clinical understanding (e.g. specialist nurse posts, academic posts).

Assignment writing

This constitutes a significant percentage of your assessment during the pre-registration programme. Some institutions try to vary the assessment strategies, not only to ease student workload but also, an assignment may not be the best way of assessing student understanding; for example, to ensure a student has the ability to supply and administer a Patient Group Direction may be best assessed using an objective structured clinical examination (OSCE) format rather than a written assignment. When writing an assignment, however, there are a number of issues and points to consider, some of which are covered below (see Chapter 6 for further guidance).

There are also a number of texts available to help you to improve your presentations. Being able to reference accurately is a good start and *Cite them Right* by Pears and Shields (2013) is a good place to start for referencing help.

The question

Take care to examine the question you are answering. The lecturers have an idea about what they want you to investigate, discuss and think about through your academic writing. You need to be clear about what this is or it could result in you producing a good piece of work but one that does not address the assignment brief and, at worst, results in a referral. Referrals in the last year of a nursing programme can cause great stress at a time when you already have anxieties relating to your transition but more importantly this has a significant impact on your final classification. Seeking academic support is recommended to ensure that you have understood the aims of the assignment and how it should be presented. Even if you think you know what they want and have always done well before, complacency at this point in your programme could have detrimental consequences. A 15-minute tutorial is not going to take too much out of your busy schedule and could give you some useful advice that could help the assignment progress much quicker.

Webb (2011) suggests that there are clear outcomes that should be identifiable within a research question. These are:

- *Descriptors* like 'describe' or 'discuss', and you may be guided at what level to do this; 'critical discussion', which is more likely to be asked of you in the second or third year of your programme.
- *The topic* – what is it about (e.g. heart failure)?
- *Context* (e.g. examining the management of any issues, examining research).

You also need to identify the presentation guidelines; for example, do they want it in a report format or is it a reflective assignment? Generally, the assignment question should indicate whether they are asking you to 'reflect,' 'report on' or 'critically anal-yse'. The latter would suggest that this is a straightforward critical discussion with no specific guidance and requirement other than academic level. A report is different because it will need separate sections and will have a specific format that you may want to check out with your tutor. Things like the structure, sections to be included and recommendations can all help to ensure you produce a report that addresses the brief required. A report will also need a clear index for easy reference. On the other hand, if it is a reflective piece you will need to identify the reflective model adopted for the work and why you selected that particular model.

Resources to help you produce a good grade are worth looking at. Your librarian at the institution you are based will have specific core texts to help support you. When performing a literature review – for example, having two or three research textbooks to refer to in your assignment – can help you clarify what you mean by the research terms. Books surrounding how to write your literature review can also be helpful. If it is a report, the Department of Health (DH) (1999) generally provides policies in report format so this may give you an indication surrounding the layout expected. If in doubt, ask!

Example assignment plan

This is an example of how a plan may look and what you may need to include. It is not meant to be prescriptive but should give you some ideas about constructing your assignment.

Assignment title
A written report critically discussing a defined public health campaign.

In this assignment you need to identify the 'defined' public health campaign: did you select it or did the tutors select it? It requires critical analysis and it should be presented as a report. It is important that it logically progresses, as a report needs to have a clear route through the subject matter.

The introduction
Briefly introduce the campaign to the reader and give reasons for selecting it if this was your choice of campaigns.

Main body
This is the discussion section of your work. This is where you need to ensure that there is criticality in your work as it is explicit in the title that you should 'critically discuss', so rather than simply saying 'Brown states this and Smith states that', try to rationalize the reasons for the differing opinion or if they have a similar opinion, are there any alternatives?

At this point you may describe the campaign in more detail than you did in the introduction. You may identify why the campaign is needed and who it is targeted at? What are the potential issues in targeting those individuals? Are there any groups that need including but may be difficult to reach with this campaign? Are there any other campaigns that are similar, and what are the advantages and limitations of those campaigns? You may need to address the health promotion models utilized within the campaigns and suggest alternatives.

Conclusion

This is a section that is undervalued but it is often the last thing read. It needs to draw together the points you have made throughout the work. If you do not have a separate recommendation section, you need to address 'what next?' How are you going to take this forward? What does it all mean?

Recommendations

This is important in a report and really for level 6 writing, it demonstrates key understanding of issues with the ability to solve problems and address those issues. It is the final section where you make recommendations for future practice including evaluation of the campaign. In this section you may want to answer the following questions rather than in the conclusion: 'What next?' How are you going to take this forward? What does it all mean?

Criticality

This is a term that may raise anxiety for some students. They may ask repeatedly, 'Am I being critical enough?' The reason we want you to be critical is to allow you to demonstrate your understanding and to use your voice in your writing. You have experience and knowledge and should be able to identify the impact this has on practice and how it could be improved.

Case study 2.1 illustrates how to take forward an observation or finding and analyse what it could mean for practice, which you will need to do if you are thinking critically.

Case study 2.1: Lisa

Lisa is undertaking a literature review examining chronic obstructive pulmonary disease (COPD) and its impact on psychological well-being. She has determined that the participants in all the studies feel socially and emotionally isolated. When discussing this with her tutor she was unsure how to proceed. They had a discussion. The tutor asked her what that meant for patients with COPD. She said that clearly they felt socially and emotionally isolated so they may need more support. The tutor agreed and asked, 'So what does that mean for the service we currently offer?' She replied stating that it may not meet patients' needs if these studies are generalizable. The tutor agreed and they followed this with a discussion regarding what they could offer that may address this deficit. Lisa was left feeling more confident about her direction but also about her ability to see the problem and solve it.

Overly descriptive or lacks criticality

You may have seen this on your assignment feedback. This is when you have simply reproduced what the evidence states but in your own words or you have not introduced any evidence at all. This demonstrates only that you can rewrite work and pull out relevant information from your background reading or that you are relying heavily on your own anecdotal experience. Evidence has a hierarchy (Wright and Ferns, 2010) and in academic writing, more credible evidence (i.e. primary research, systematic reviews, discussion articles that have been peer reviewed and presented in academic journals or textbooks) would be appropriate to refer to. Referencing this varied material would exhibit an in-depth understanding as you would be demonstrating that you have examined a range of evidence. This is what is required of you at level 6. It is about taking ideas forward and not simply stating what authors suggest (see the example assignment above). It is about asking 'so what?' What is happening in this situation? What does this mean to practice? What could we do about this?

If you have a paragraph that has no references included in it, then this should ring alarm bells. It may mean that you are just telling a story or giving your interpretation. Perhaps you do need to refer to a practice situation but that needs to be linked to the evidence you are citing and it should not be an extensive description.

Theory and practice

Lecturers may continually discuss links between theory and practice. This is not a requirement that comes simply from the academic environment. It has been established through research and through practice reviews that, for a nurse to be fit for practice, they need to be able to understand the theory that underpins their practice. This theoretical understanding should underpin your decision-making processes and you should be able to discuss the rationale.

The standards for pre-registration education require this and suggest that the ability to not only understand the theoretical evidence but also being able to appraise it is paramount for safe and effective nursing practice. On entering the register you remain bound to practice using the best available evidence (NMC, 2015) that again highlights the requirement for the link. Standing (2011) suggests that it is not simply a case of linking theory to practice but this process should involve an examination of our personal experience of the event, situation or case, recognizing the importance to be able to learn from it.

It is important that you continually strive to bridge the gaps between theory and practice that still exist despite the changes in nursing curricula (UKCC, 1986; NMC, 2010). These gaps present newly qualified nurses (NQNs) with significant challenges and result in great anxiety both nationally and internationally as shown in studies by Havn and Vedi (1997) and Odland et al. (2014). Despite the vast difference in year of publication of the studies, 1997 and 2014, this theory–practice gap remained evident in both. Clearly applying your theoretical knowledge and reflecting upon it but also recalling it in new situations all form part of the learning experience. It may be that the assignment that links theory to practice is the start of the learning experience, and when the topic of the assignment has been experienced again in practice and the theory recalled, a further consolidation of your learning could result. Although this discussion does not help you write at level 6, it does highlight the importance for you as a student nurse to relate theory to practice as you are about to embark on a career as a qualified nurse.

Peer support

Using your peers during background reading and tutorials can be helpful (Gopee and Deane, 2013). Discussing the assignment and issues relating to the topic area can help with understanding and give new perspectives. It may also incite motivation and enthusiasm as areas where there is some misunderstanding could be addressed in a safe environment; that is, among friends or peers that one may feel comfortable with.

Reflection

Think of a difficult task you have experienced, for example, stopping smoking, going on a diet, going to see the bank! Did you have support and was this helpful? If you did not, do you think it would have been helpful to have had some support?

In academic writing, support can have a great impact on your ability to achieve a very positive outcome. Working together may strengthen your ability to carry on with the same enthusiasm as you started with or instigate some enthusiasm if deficient due to lack of understanding in the initial stages. Gopee and Deane (2013) identified in their research, when examining successful strategies for academic writing, that this supportive approach empowered individuals as it appears to be a proactive means of study. The participants also referred to the adage that 'two heads are better than one' so when you are in a tutorial, your peers may ask a question that you had not considered, which may help give your assignment a different dimension or prompt greater depth within your discussion.

There is a suggestion that this may be further enhanced by peer review of your assignment (Rieber, 2006). Rieber (2006) compared the academic attainment of business students. He had two groups: one group was allocated peer reviewing and the second group had conventional support, that is, no peer review was instigated. The peer review group had significantly higher grades. Rieber (2006) identified potential reasons for this and all seem feasible but also they seem desirable. Suggested reasons offered included early completion to take into account the review process and possible amendment time required, and taking greater care over their work as they are aware that their peers are reviewing therefore wanting to appear more intelligent or competent. Anxieties with this process could involve the chances of plagiarism but all students are aware that work is submitted through plagiarism software therefore this should prevent an academic offence such as this. In fact, it may be that it dissuades students from plagiarism as they may seek greater support from their peers.

Conclusion

This chapter has emphasized that seeking support adds to the clarity needed in order to maximize your potential for successful writing at level 6. We have also seen that planning your work and examining what the question is asking of you is vital to ensure you address the question fully. Level 6 writing requires a problem-solving approach so it means unpicking and examining what the evidence implies and questioning it, perhaps proposing alternative options or conclusions. Finally, linking theory to practice is not just an exercise that the NMC (2010) states you should do but can help you in the future when embarking on the transition from student to qualified nurse.

References

Department of Health (DH) (1999) *Health Service Circular – Making a Difference to Nursing and Midwifery Pre-registration Education.* HSC 1999/219, 1–18. London: Her Majesty's Stationery Office (HMSO).

Gonzales, J. and Wagenaar, R. (2003) *Tuning Educational Structures in Europe: Final Report Pilot Project-Phase 1.* Bilbao: University of Deusto.

Gopee, N. and Deane, M. (2013) Strategies for successful academic writing: institutional and non-institutional support for students, *Nurse Education Today*, 33(12): 1624–1631.

Havn, V. and Vedi, C. (1997) *PÅ DYPT VANN – Om nyutdannede sykepleieres kompetanse i møte med en somatisk sengepost [On Newly Qualified Nurses' Competence in Encounters with a General Ward]. Report.* Trondheim, Norway: SINTEF-group.

Maben, J. and Macleod Clarke, J. (1998) Project 2000 diplomats' perceptions of their experiences of transition from student to staff nurse, *Journal of Clinical Nursing*, 7(2): 145–153.

Nursing and Midwifery Council (NMC) (2010) *Standards for Pre-Registration Nursing Education.* London: NMC.

Nursing and Midwifery Council (NMC) (2015) *The Code: Professional Standards of Practice and Behaviour for Nurses and Midwives.* London: NMC.

Odland, L., Sneltvedt, T. and Sorlie, V. (2014) Responsible but unprepared: experiences of newly educated nurses in hospital care, *Nurse Education in Practice*, 14(5): 538–543.

Pears, R. and Shields, G. (2013) *Cite them Right: The Essential Referencing Guide*, 9th edn. Basingstoke: Palgrave.

Rieber, L. J. (2006) Using peer review to improve student writing in business course, *Journal of Business Education*, March/April, 322–326.

Standing, M. (2011) *Clinical Judgement and Decision Making for Student Nurses.* London: Learning Matters.

United Kingdom Central Council (UKCC) for Nursing and Midwifery (1986) *Project 2000: A New Preparation for Practice.* London: UKCC.

Webb, L. (2011) *Nursing: Communication Skills in Practice.* Oxford: Oxford University Press.

Wright, K. and Ferns, T. (2010) Simple writing skills for students part two: researching your subject, *British Journal of Nursing*, 19(17): 1118–1120.

3 Evidence-based practice for the newly qualified nurse

Overview

All students on nursing degree programmes will have been exposed to the concept of evidence-based practice (EBP) before they reach their third year. This chapter begins with some revision of the subject. However, the main focus is on how and why this will become important in your final year in practice and in your first year as a newly qualified nurse (NQN). This includes advice on constructing your own research project as well as examining others' evidence base for practice. Finally, this chapter provides advice on how to indicate expertise in EBP to your lecturers.

Introduction

Throughout your nursing programme and your career as a registered nurse (RN) you must demonstrate that you are basing your practice on the best available evidence. In your first two years as a student you will have studied the basic components of ensuring an evidence base for nursing. In the third year you will be expected to demonstrate your ability to critically analyse the best evidence for practice. Many courses will have a research-based dissertation or long essay. The purpose of this is to ensure that students can understand the research process to the extent of designing and possibly implementing a systematic review or a small research project. Consequently, this chapter begins by briefly revisiting the research process which is essential knowledge for nurses to decide what the best evidence for practice is. Following this, it considers how and why EBP will be important in your final year as a student and when you start as an NQN.

Revision of EBP

Evidence-based practice (EBP) is a problem-solving approach to clinical care that incorporates the conscientious use of current best evidence from well-designed studies, a clinician's expertise, and patient values and preferences.

Meinyk and Fineout-Overholt (2005)

Evidence-based nursing can be defined as the application of valid, relevant, research-based information in nurse decision-making.

Cullum *et al.* (2008)

Using EBP is common sense and most of the general public would be surprised that healthcare professionals would consider looking after them in any other way.

It is simply ensuring that we are providing the best care according to the current evidence available. Of course, in order for nurses to be able to provide the best care in a rapidly progressing evidence-based environment, they must be able to understand the research process that produces the evidence. The reason why it is important for nurses to understand research is that otherwise you have no way of working out which way of doing things is the best. Case study 3.1 illustrates this problem.

Case study 3.1: Research has shown . . .

You have just started a new placement and your mentor tells you that the manual handling technique that you've been taught in university is old fashioned and dangerous. You check the procedure guide for the placement and it says that the technique you have been taught is correct. Being a brave third year, you bring this up with your mentor at the first opportunity. He laughs and says: 'Yes, but the hospital policy is out of date too. Research has shown that the way we do it here is better for the nurse and the patient.' He then produces a research paper that he suggests you read. You quickly see that the findings of the researchers agree with your mentor that the new way is better.

Reflection

- Does this prove that your mentor's manual handling method is the best evidence-based way?
- How can you check that this is right or wrong?
- If you are convinced that the new manual handling technique is evidence-based will you use it even though it contradicts the hospital policy?

You may think that the best thing to do is to ask someone in authority. For example, you may ask the matron on your placement or one of your lecturers. They may be able to provide you with some insight and may have already looked into this issue. Another option is to simply follow the procedure manual or the university's teaching as they are both likely to have been considered at length by senior nurses and selected as the best methods. Nonetheless, things change rapidly in healthcare and to gain solid evidence you need to search the research literature that exists on the subject.

The most important thing to know is that there are hierarchies of evidence. In other words, depending on what it is that you want to look into, different sources of evidence are seen as more reliable. As can be seen from Box 3.1, systematic reviews are considered the best source of evidence. This is because they bring together all of the evidence collected in primary research. Consequently, they are much more reliable than a single research project report.

Box 3.1: Hierarchy of evidence sources

1. Systematic review or meta-analysis of randomized control trials (RCTs).
2. RCTs.
3. Systematic reviews of double blind peer-reviewed research other than RCTs.
4. Double blind peer-reviewed research other than RCTs.
5. Authoritative reports based on expert opinion.

If you are trying to find out whether the results of a research report like the one in Case study 3.1 are right, then the best way is to find or create a systematic review of all of the evidence on the subject. With the easy access that students and health workers now have to research databases, this is entirely possible. The usual advice on searching the literature is to conduct logical systematic search strategies. There are recognized checklists to help you to formulate a search strategy and to justify your results such as the 'Preferred Reporting Items for Systematic Reviews and Meta-Analyses (PRISMA)' (Blegen, 2010). This checklist works best with RCTs but can be used as a framework for constructing systematic reviews of other kinds of research. However, if you are seeking evidence to support your practice, perhaps to use as an argument to support a particular form of practice, then a straightforward logical approach such as the following systematic approach (Aveyard, 2014) should be sufficient.

1. Decide what you are looking for.
2. Select the database to search.
3. Decide on keywords to enter into your database.
4. Decide on limiters such as language, chronology and geographical location.
5. Conduct the search.
6. Select the appropriate articles by reading titles, abstracts and finally full articles.
7. Create a table with the findings and limitations of each article listed.
8. Discuss the findings and limitations of the articles.
9. Synthesize your discussion into a conclusion.
10. Recommend actions for practice and future research.

These will be expanded upon using the research subject of preceptorship for NQNs as an example to illustrate the steps.

Step 1 is the most important and needs some careful thought. Once you have decided on the subject you will need to follow the list to the end to find your answer.

Step 2 is all about working out where to look for the evidence. Specialist nursing databases are available through hospital libraries for staff and university libraries for students. Librarians are often skilled in searching databases and will help you if you ask the right questions. The most important thing is to have a clear idea of what you are looking for. Databases are collections of journals selected to meet the needs of specific users. Two examples of those serving nurses are the Cumulative Index to Nursing and Allied Health Literature (CINAHL) and the British Nursing Index (BNI). These are a good way of selecting only articles from nursing and allied health journals and therefore mean that you do not have to sift out all of the usual unreliable sources that can be found by standard web search engines such as Google or Bing. An intermediary way of searching for evidence is using internet search engines that are designed to find authoritative academic articles such as Google Scholar and PubMed. It is often useful to search one of these at the beginning in order to quickly see if there is anything available on the subject that you are interested in. It is often possible to find an existing published systematic review on the issue you are researching. If it is a good one, you may not need to look any further. Other good sources of existing systematic reviews are databases purely of systematic reviews of the literature that fit a prescribed set of criteria. Two of the most well known are the Cochrane and Joanna Briggs Institute libraries of systematic reviews. These are best for literature reviews of RCTs and are medically focused. Consequently, the best database to use depends on what it is that you are looking for.

Step 3: the way that databases know what you want to search for is by you adding keywords to their search boxes. The keywords you use should be carefully chosen based upon the subject that you are trying to find out about. Two established methods of selecting keywords are known as PICO and SPICE.

PICO

P **Patient or population**
I **Intervention**
C **Comparator**
O **Outcomes**

SPICE

S **Setting** – Where? In what context?
P **Perspective** – For who?
I **Intervention** (Phenomenon of Interest) – What?
C **Comparison** – What else?
E **Evaluation** – How well? What result?

PICO works best with searches for medical treatments and SPICE is best for more social phenomena such as how best to run a ward, or how to improve preceptorship programmes for NQNs. However, they can be used interchangeably depending on what is being searched for, and the one that fits best is the right one.

Step 4: limitations to your search can be useful if there is a lot of evidence or if your interest is specific to a region or country. If you are using a chronological limitation, it is best practice to think of a reason to start your search at a particular year rather than to select a year at random. For example, when investigating preceptorship for NQNs you could use 1990, which was the first time that preceptorship was advised by the United Kingdom Central Council for Nursing,

Midwifery and Health Visiting (UKCC, 1990), or 2010, which was when the Department of Health laid out its standards for preceptorship (DH, 2010).

Step 5 is to conduct the search. You may think that this is a simple matter of inputting the information you have collected in steps 2 to 4. In essence, it is, but it may not be that simple. Until you run the search you will not know if the search criteria will bring out anything sensible. It could generate hundreds of thousands of hits or, at the other extreme, none. If either of these things happens you will need to refine your search criteria. It may take several attempts to generate a sensible number of articles. In addition to this mechanical search, you can also look at the reference lists of the ones you have found.

Step 6 involves selecting the most appropriate articles from those that you have found to read and critically analyse. The best way to do this is to read the titles and reject anything that does not fit your need for research articles. Consequently, anything that is an editorial, a news report, letter to the editor, book review or a 'how to do it' article should be rejected. You should then have a selection of research articles that appear to be relevant. The next step is to read their abstracts to see if they fit the criteria. Those that fit the criteria should be read in their entirety. If you are doing this to simply find out for yourself if a research report is in line with the current state-of-the-art thinking on the subject, then this will probably satisfy you at this stage. However, if you are writing a report to try to convince other professionals, such as your mentor, the matron or your lecturer, then you will be best advised to complete steps 7–10 as well. These are also necessary if you are writing an article or meeting the criteria of a systematic literature review assignment for your course.

Step 7 is to create a table with the findings and limitations of each article listed. The table of articles can be as simple or as complex as you like. In its most basic form you simply need to list the articles, the method used to collect the data, including the number of participants, and the findings.

Step 8 is the most important as you will discuss and interpret the findings presented in the table. The usual way to present the discussion is by selecting themes that emerge from the findings that you have described in step 7. These themes may not have been evident to the original researchers but come out of the process of reading all of the research output on the issue. Therefore, this is where you add something new to the critical analysis of the subject.

Step 9 provides you with the opportunity to describe briefly the main points of your discussion. You should not add anything new to this stage as you are bringing together everything you have found out.

Step 10: finally and most importantly, you need to put forward your recommendations for practice and future research. In the case of a specific manual handling procedure it may be that you recommend its use, or that you recommend it is not used or that another procedure is preferable. Whichever it is should clearly follow from the evidence you have presented. Your recommendations for future research should suggest where the gaps are in what has been done already or where existing research needs to be repeated in order to strengthen its reliability and show that it is repeatable.

How and why EBP will become important in your final year in practice as a student

As indicated in the previous section, you may well be required to write a literature review following a systematic approach similar to the one described above. If not, then using this method to analyse and criticize evidence will be invaluable in both the theory and practice components of your course. By your final year of the programme you will be expected to be able to assess the evidence for anything that you are involved with in order to work out if it is the best EBP for your patients.

Reflection

Use Case study 3.1 at the beginning of the chapter for the reflections below.

- Hospital policies would usually be considered to fit into the hierarchy of evidence above at the bottom of the list. However, it may be that the experts who have compiled it based their opinion upon systematic reviews or other research. How could you check this?
- In your transition from student to RN, it is likely that you will come across competing sources of evidence. Policies and procedure guides such as the one discussed in Case study 3.1 are designed to be evidence based and to ensure that everyone is caring for their patients in the same way. Can you think of a reason why it may sometimes be best to ensure that everyone follows the same procedure, until the policy is officially reviewed, even if it has been superseded by the evidence?

In your assignments in your final year, if you refer to the evidence analysis methods and discussions about best practice indicated in the 10-step systematic approach to evidence selection and analysis above, you will be critically analysing the arguments presented at a higher level. This is generally seen as a good thing by academic assessors. Consequently, even if you are not conducting a systematic review, it is ideal to show that you have knowledge of these skills in your academic writing as well as using them in your clinical practice.

How and why EBP will become important in your first year as an NQN

In your first year as a qualified nurse the ability to examine the evidence for each activity will be invaluable. You will be anxious to ensure that you are doing your best for your patients. The fact is that examining and carefully interpreting the evidence base for your practice is the only way to ensure that you are doing your best for your patients within the context of the healthcare system.

EBP is important at every stage of a nurse's career. However, in the final stage of the pre-registration course and in the first year after qualifying, it is most acutely necessary to have the skills to work out what is the best practice for your patients. In earlier stages of your course you are learning these skills and later in your career you will have amassed a great deal of practical and theoretical experience. Therefore, learning and utilizing research and analysis skills is extremely important during this period of transition from student to qualified nurse.

References

Aveyard, H. (2014) *Doing a Literature Review in Health and Social Care: A Practical Guide*, 3rd edn. Maidenhead: Open University Press.

Blegen, M. A. (2010) Editorial: PRISMA, *Nursing Research*, 59(4): 233.

Cullum, N., Ciliska, D., Haynes, B. and Marks, S. (2008) *Evidence-based Nursing: An Introduction*. Oxford: Blackwell.

Department of Health (DH) (2010) *Preceptorship Framework for Newly Registered Nurses, Midwives and Allied Health Professionals*. London: DH.

Melnyk, B. and Fineout-Overholt, E. (2005) Transforming healthcare from the inside out: advancing evidence based practice in the 21st century, *Journal of Professional Nursing*, 21(6): 335–344.

United Kingdom Central Council (UKCC) for Nursing, Midwifery and Health Visiting (1990) *The Report of the Post-registration Education and Practice Project*. London: UKCC.

4 Leadership and delegation in nursing

Overview

Theories of leadership and management are likely to figure in the learning and assessment process of nursing programmes. This chapter examines some of the central themes in these with a view to outlining their usefulness to your practice. It also gives practical advice on providing evidence to your lecturers that these concepts have been understood.

Introduction

As you approach the end of the final year of your nursing programme, you must demonstrate a level of competency and skill in managing patient care. The skill required at your level should include an ability to delegate, co-ordinate and maintain patient safety. Once you have demonstrated this, you will then be acknowledged as fit for practice at the point of registration. This is deemed to be a safe standard and level of knowledge in which to practise as a newly qualified staff nurse. You should be prepared to demonstrate your skills in this area of leadership and delegation when you are assessed in practice in order to show you meet the requisite level of competency to achieve Nursing and Midwifery Council (NMC) domains. However, managing, delegating and leading a team is not merely a practical skill: your ability to understand the theoretical underpinnings surrounding management and leadership is vital in order for you to be able to adapt your leadership and management styles according to the situation you are in.

This may be an anxious time as although delegation and management will have been an element of your role over your time in the programme, it may have been quite discreet, without too much emphasis and close scrutiny. Now it will be examined as part of your performance. What one should be mindful of is that you have gained a vast amount of experience over the last three years, which will inform your decisions and allow you to make what are, often, very good decisions. You will already be able to think of occasions when you have had to support your decision-making process and give a clear rationale for them in previous placements and in the academic environment, and this will be an important element in your final year. The following case studies demonstrate how decision-making skills can enhance the clinical environment and how leading a team can help to increase patient safety and enhance a team approach.

Case study 4.1: Rita

Rita is in charge of the Accident and Emergency (A&E) department. They have just had a call to warn them of a serious road traffic accident involving a number of casualties, some of whom require intensive assessment and treatment. Their estimated time of arrival is 10 minutes. Rita responds quickly, calling her staff. She allocates staff to treatment and resuscitation rooms. She tells them what they need to do and to keep her informed of the patients that attend. She wants half-hourly updates of the situation but if there is anything urgent, then they are to seek her advice immediately. She telephones the anaesthetist and asks him to come to A&E and informs the consultant that more medical staff will be required in the department in the next five minutes.

Reflection

- How would you feel in this situation?
- Do you think the nurse's autocratic style is appropriate, and if so why?
- If you were a member of Rita's team, could she have asked your opinion or asked you which area you would rather be in? If not, why?

Case study 4.2: Laura

Laura was in charge of a group of Macmillan nurses. Each had worked in the department for between 5 and 10 years. Laura was new to the team and insisted on delegating all new referrals and wanted feedback on a daily basis about the patient contacts. In addition, she wanted weekly written reports. In the daily feedbacks she proceeded to tell the staff what she would have done, which was often different to what the nurses had actually carried out.

Reflection

- Laura has the same autocratic approach to the A&E nurse. Do you think it is appropriate?
- If you do not, why not?
- Is there a more appropriate way to liaise with her staff?

Leading and managing a team needs a great deal of consideration as it can be a complex situation or one where time to consider the alternatives is limited. One may argue that being responsive to situations, adapting to changes is common-place in the healthcare environment. If we think of a situation like a nurse in charge dealing with a cardiac arrest on a ward, they may need to adopt an auto-cratic approach rather than their usual style where they ask staff's opinions or for their contribution to any decision making. Having an understanding surrounding your teams and the individual staffs' needs and concerns can all help to create a harmonious, supportive and enthusiastic team because the staff may feel valued and invested in. A manager who lacks any awareness of a low morale in their staff, or conflict, or even, at worst, bullying, loses respect and may find an increase in staff turnover. Not only does this place a great deal of burden upon the staff members but it may have an impact on patient care. As a nurse who has had placements in a variety of clinical areas, you may recall some excellent leaders and managers.

Reflection

We have mentioned 'the team' several times. It may be worth examining the concept of the team. Bach and Ellis (2011) determined that to ensure a positive working environment and effective team dynamics, the team itself should know exactly what the objectives are, have positive relationships and feel supported. In addition, a spirit of collaboration and co-operation in the pursuit of the aims and goals will help the team to achieve those goals.

Reflection

- Think about the placements you have had. Think especially of the team leaders you have worked with.
- Can you recall the qualities in the leader that inspired you?
- Think about how you could adopt some of these qualities in your leadership role.
- Have you experienced any areas where the team leader seemed to have difficulties with their team?
- What do you think went wrong in those situations?
- How have you contributed to teams and teamwork?
- What motivated you to work within the team or teams?
- List the effective and not so effective team characteristics you have experienced.

Yoder-Wise (2015) identified a number of characteristics that may influence the success or failure of a team to work in a cohesive manner. These characteristics range from the environment, including whether it is strained or supportive, and open, to the way in which the team contribute to decision making or receive feedback from tasks carried out or ideas suggested.

Ultimately, we all want to feel supported, valued and included. This may help to create a more harmonious team where there is a supportive atmosphere and a camaraderie that inspires and motivates a team to want to provide excellent care while ensuring that there is a compassionate and caring approach to all team members too.

Belbin (2010) identified a number of roles that people may adopt when in a team. He suggests that individuals tend to be dominant in one or two team roles but can adopt roles or elements of a role that may be missing in a team in order for it to function. Belbin's work derives from his research surrounding dysfunctional teams in the 1970s and suggests there are nine key team roles but in the absence of any one of these roles, members may need to be flexible within their team in order to incorporate the missing roles.

Case study 4.3: Group presentation

You are in your theory block and the first assessment is a group presentation. You have the learning outcomes and guidance about what you need to achieve in the presentation. You have carte blanche regarding how you present your findings. There are eight in the group. You really struggle to come up with ideas. You spend the first two sessions brainstorming the issues but still no one could identify what they should be doing or how they could present the findings.

Reflection

- What could be happening here?
- How could they overcome this?

Belbin suggests all the nine roles are required for a group to work effectively.

Belbin creates names for each role and shows their function (Belbin, 2012–14). For instance, if the 'plant', a person with imaginative ideas and problem-solving abilities, is absent in the team, then creativity may be stifled. Alternatively, if there is a lack of an 'implementer', then the ideas generated by the 'plant' may not come to fruition.

In the above scenario, the group's difficulties may be due to the absence of the 'plant' role. If the team can recognize this, then they may be able to look at their characteristics and pull on their other strengths because in actual fact each of us does not simply have to have one role in a team, we can cover two or three roles though we may have one that we perceive as more dominant (Belbin, 2012–14).

Leading rather than managing

A classic statement by Bennis (1989), who was a renowned authority surrounding leadership, still resonates today, he determined that 'leaders do the right thing' and managers 'do things right'. One may be one or both of these at the same time but it is not essential to be both. A good manager will essentially run a department as their own manager/management team requires, achieving standards as required and will follow protocol and policy in order to achieve this. A leader will try to look at the team's direction identifying future aims and challenges. They will try to inspire and be forward-thinking, developing services and asking why should we and what would happen if we did this? Leaders may be more challenging and may be identified as unique.

Leadership is an inherent part of the nursing role and within the Department of Health (DH) and the National Health Service (NHS), leadership features in standards and recommendations due to the importance it plays in the caring environment. The fact that it is acknowledged in pre-registration and post-registration educational standards emphasizes its importance for nursing progression. Specifically in your programme, tutors will ask you to demonstrate your leadership skills in group work and also in your assignments through recommendations for future practice, which should be incorporated in the conclusion for all your work, particularly in the final stage of the nursing programme.

Reflection

Think of managers you have worked with.

- Were any of them leaders too?
- If they were, what made them different and how did you feel as a team member?

Martin (2000) identifies a number of characteristics and skills that a leader may display.

- Can you list what you think they may be?

You may have come up with answers like valuing staff, motivating, making the team feel valued and giving them a voice and being innovative. This may be a list of skills but it is one that you need to be mindful of as you yourself progress in your career and have to manage or lead a team. Staff morale and teamwork are essential in the provision of high-quality nursing care but also can help staff well-being.

Linking theory to practice

Within your theory modules, your understanding surrounding leadership and management may well be questioned. What your lecturers may want to establish is not simply that you can recall a number of management models and leadership theories but that you understand how they may improve your practice as you enter the nursing register and take on the role of a qualified nurse. If you were asked to address issues like the failings at Mid Staffordshire (Francis, 2013) as an example, your lecturer would want to see you examine the failings from a leadership and management perspective, then identify where more appropriate leadership and management techniques or models may have been beneficial. In addition, you would need to look at the theory underpinning those models. You could do this first by looking at the original sources; that is, Goleman (1998) and his work surrounding emotional intelligence in leadership and management, or Adair's (2010) action-centred leadership. Second, by looking at any research undertaken that has been published in reputable nursing and healthcare journals as well as (third) addressing policy and standards for management and leadership; for example, the NHS Leadership Academy (2013). You should examine the evidence and apply that knowledge of the theory and policy and standards to the practice situation. You could then identify how this could improve the practice and suggest who it would benefit.

Delegation

Part of your role as a qualified nurse will be to work in a team and delegate to members of that team on a regular basis. Delegation is a way of empowering the team rather than marginalizing them and doing everything yourself. The Code (NMC, 2015) states that delegation is paramount within your roles and responsibilities. Gill (2011) suggests that delegation that is done to develop people empowers, but in a healthcare environment workload and time management are often the factors that influence the decision to delegate. Whatever the reason, its benefits may be numerous with minimal disadvantages. Those disadvantages could be surrounding the delegator's responsibility to check that the task or duty has been done correctly, and this may be quite time consuming, or there may be some reluctance by the delegatee to perform the task and this may cause frustration, but generally, these are minimal when compared to the clear benefits such as helping people to develop their competency and confidence. Investing in the development of colleagues is, once again, a requirement that is advocated by the NMC (2015) therefore supporting people in undertaking tasks and other responsibilities is essential. This philosophy of sharing responsibility can aid a more collegiate and effective team approach to patient care and facilitate development within the team.

Teamworking in the healthcare environment is vital for safe and effective patient care and for the well-being of staff in the environment. As Finkleman (2012) states, 'no one can do it all'. What you should remember is that you have been working in a team all the way through your nursing programme so continuing to do this in the final part of your programme, and when you become a qualified nurse, should not present you with undue stress. When you qualify you may feel more anxiety about being part of a team because you are going to be part of an established team and may want to feel valued within that team therefore the way you fit in and integrate may be more important to you. Effective teamworking is not just important to you; however, Belbin (2010) identified that dysfunctional teamworking can cause a number of problems. If we apply this to the healthcare environment, a team that fails to communicate effectively, support each other or be compassionate with each other may provide ineffective, poor quality care that fails to meet patients' needs and lacks the compassionate approach we should be providing.

Conclusion

Your final year is an opportunity to consolidate the knowledge and skills you have developed and attained over the last few years to help inform your practice and manage and lead others in delivering high-quality care. Delegation and leadership are not just requisites of a qualified nurse. There is a requirement for you, as a student nurse, to develop the confidence and ability to lead and delegate as well as manage, but also, this is a really good opportunity that will help you to prepare for your future role as a staff nurse. Considering the leadership and management qualities you have witnessed in your career to date, which may include experience that pre-dates your student nurse role, can help you to identify the type of leader you want to be and to learn from the success of others. Reflect and harness that experience to help you support and achieve excellence within your team.

References

Adair, J. (2010) *Develop your Leadership Skills*. London: Kogan Page.

Bach, S. and Ellis, P. (2011) *Leadership, Management, and Team Working in Nursing*. Exeter: Learning Matters.

Belbin, M. R. (2010) *Managing Teams: Why they Succeed or Fail*, 3rd edn. Oxford: Butterworth Heinemann.

Belbin, M. R (2012–14) *Belbin Team Roles*. Available at: http://www.belbin.com/rte.asp?id=8 (accessed: 17 September 2015).

Bennis, W. G. (1989) *On Becoming a Leader*. New York: Addison Wesley.

Finkleman, A. (2012) *Leadership and Management for Nurses: Core Competencies for Quality Care*, 2nd edn. Hoboken, NJ: Pearson.

Francis, R. (2013) *Report of the Mid Staffordshire NHS Foundation Trust Public Inquiry*. London: Her Majesty's Stationery Office (HMSO).

Gill, G. (2011) *Theory and Practice of Leadership*, 2nd edn. London: Sage.

Goleman, D. (1998) *Working with Emotional Intelligence*. New York: Bantam Books.

Martin, V. (2000) Effective team leadership, *Nursing Management*, 10(5): 26–29.

NHS Leadership Academy (2013) *Healthcare Leadership Model*. Leeds: NHS Leadership Academy. Available at: http://www.leadershipacademy.nhs.uk/wp-content/uploads/dlm_uploads/2014/10/NHSLeadership-LeadershipModel-colour.pdf (accessed: 17 September 2015).

Nursing and Midwifery Council (NMC) (2015) *The Code*. London: NMC.

Yoder-Wise, P. S. (2015) *Leading and Managing In Nursing*, 6th ed. St Louis, MO: Elsevier Mosby.

5 | Teaching for the newly qualified nurse

Overview

From the point of registration, all nurses are required to have a teaching element to their role. It is essential therefore for the final year student to learn about the theories and practice of education related to nursing. This chapter outlines these theories in a similar way to the chapter dealing with leadership theory.

Introduction

The Nursing and Midwifery Council (NMC) requires nurses at the point of registration to be able to teach both patients and other nurses. This is supported by the NMC Standards to Support Learning and Assessment in Practice (NMC, 2008) and the NMC Code (NMC, 2015). Both of these documents make it clear that all nurses must 'support students' and colleagues' learning to help them develop their professional competence and confidence' (NMC, 2015: 9). Further underlining this expectation is the statement that 'the NMC would expect that the majority of nurses and midwives would at least meet the outcomes of a mentor' (NMC, 2008: 19). Therefore, the regulatory framework for nurses is very clear that they must be teachers as well as carers.

However, even if this were not so, it is evident that teaching students and patients is central to the role of the nurse. Nurses learn at least half of their skills in the clinical area. Professional nurse teachers and practice teachers support this learning but the majority of everyday teaching in practice is done by registered nurses (RNs). Nurses also have to teach patients and carers. This includes topics such as: how to use an inhaler; how to care for their wound dressing; how to self-inject; how to use continence products; pelvic floor exercises; and so many others that it would be impractical to list them all. In addition, nurses support teaching by physicians and allied health professions such as physiotherapists and speech and language therapists.

Consequently, as a nurse, you will need to have an understanding of the fundamentals of teaching and learning theory. Some of the important structures of education are now outlined, followed by how they can be used in practice and ways of providing evidence to your lecturers of your level of understanding.

Learn about the theories and practice of education related to nursing

Education is a profession with a similar level of theoretical underpinning to the profession of nurses. As a nurse you are not expected to become an education professional unless you become a nurse teacher. However, as indicated above, you will need to understand the fundamental underpinnings of educational theory. This is a topic around which there is a lot of debate, and the theories and frameworks put forward here are a selection. However, this will give you a start in this field.

Educational taxonomies

Taxonomies are systems of naming or classifying things. Therefore, educational taxonomies are attempting to name the different components of the process of learning and teaching. The most well known and most often referred to of these is Bloom's taxonomy (Bloom, 1956; Anderson *et al.*, 2001). There are two main components to Bloom's taxonomy. The first is the idea that there are domains of learning and the second component is a hierarchy of learning within each domain.

The domains are described as indicated in Box 5.1.

Box 5.1: The domains of learning

- Cognitive domain: knowledge
- Affective domain: attitudes
- Psychomotor domain: skills

As can be seen in Box 5.1 this is an attempt to split up learning into different ways in which we use our brains. All three domains are important in nursing. The cognitive domain has most often been focused on by educationalists because it describes the traditional higher education subjects. However, in nursing the emotions encompassed in the affective domain and the physical skills in the psychomotor domain are equally important.

The hierarchies of learning within each domain have been developed in the 60 years since Bloom's taxonomy was first published and the latest versions are used below (Krathwohl *et al.*, 1964; Dave, 1970).

The bullet point at the top of each list is considered to be the most advanced but is built upon the hierarchy of bullet points below it.

Cognitive domain: knowledge

- Creating
- Evaluating
- Analysing
- Applying

- Understanding
- Remembering

Affective domain: attitudes

- Characterizing by value
- Organizing and conceptualizing
- Valuing
- Responding
- Receiving

Psychomotor domain: skills

- Naturalization
- Articulation
- Precision
- Manipulation
- Imitation

There are also other taxonomies such as the Structure of the Observed Learning Outcome (SOLO) taxonomy devised by Biggs (Biggs and Tang, 2011), who describes this as:

> At first we pick up only one or few aspects of the task (unistructural), then several aspects but they are unrelated (multistructural), then we learn how to integrate them into a whole (relational), and finally, we are able to generalise that whole to as yet untaught applications (extended abstract).
>
> Biggs (n.d.)

This is illustrated in the following list:

- extended abstract: theorizes and reflects
- relational: compares and contrasts
- multistructural: combines procedures
- unistructural: identifies how to do a simple procedure
- prestructural: misses the point.

> Biggs and Tang (2011)

Benner described a similar process in a nursing context. She described this as the progression from novice to expert that she believed was a journey that every excellent nurse took in their career (Benner, 1984). The stages are as follows:

- novice
- advanced beginner
- competent
- proficient
- expert.

She argued that progression through the stages is not a natural result of 'the passage of time or longevity' (Benner, 1982). It is a conscious application of theory to practice over a long period of clinical experience. The nurse, as teacher, cannot only help others through these stages but can also move towards excellence, in part, by teaching others.

Teaching cycle and teaching plans

You may wish to read further on these theories but the main reason for knowing about them is to think like a teacher; that is:

- your student has a variety of things to learn
- they will learn about them in different ways depending on whether they are knowledge-based such as anatomy and physiology; emotional such as breaking bad news to a patient; or physical skills such as how to transfer a patient from a bed to a chair
- you will need to adopt different teaching strategies dependent on which of the above it is
- whatever the thing to be taught and learned is, there will be a hierarchy of learning from novice to expert.

With this in mind it is important to structure your teaching to achieve the objective; that is, the student has demonstrably learned what you wanted to teach them. The accepted way of doing this is to plan your teaching around the teaching cycle (Figure 5.1).

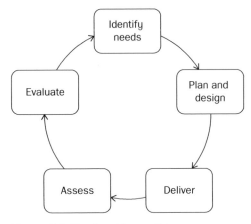

Figure 5.1 The teaching cycle

Each of these stages should be covered in your teaching plan. All teaching has to be planned and the plan should encompass all of the stages of the teaching cycle; nevertheless, the formality of the plan depends on what, when, why and for what purpose the teaching is taking place.

The teaching planner shown in Box 5.2 helps the teacher to put the plan into a formal written format. This is useful when the activity is complex; you are likely to repeat it again; or you need to provide evidence to someone else that you have conducted a good quality teaching activity. However, for most teaching activities in practice settings, the teaching plan is often less formal and just a matter of the teacher holding the stages of the teaching cycle in their mind as they teach the student. This applies unless you are a clinical nurse educator who will be required to log all of their teaching activities and provide teaching plans for monitoring purposes (Whitehead, 2010).

Box 5.2: An example teaching planner

Teaching Plan	
Session:	Location:
Date:	Time:

Learning outcomes: at the end of the session the learner will be able to demonstrate an ability to:

Time	Topic	Teacher activity	Learner activity	Resources

Method of assessment of learning:

Session evaluation:

Using theories in practice

Case study 5.1 illustrates how some of the themes from the education theories can be used in practice.

Case study 5.1: Bed bath

A first-year student has been asked to give a patient a bed bath for the first time. You are supervising her doing this at the request of her mentor. You know that she has been taught the theory and practised the skill in clinical simulation at the university. Therefore, before you take her to the patient you ask her what she knows about the process. From her answer you plan your approach to supervising her based on the learning needs you have assessed. When you are washing the patient with her you notice that she is confident in manual handling; use of personal protective equipment; and the procedural aspects of washing the patient. However, she is only speaking to you rather than the patient and although you talk to the patient throughout she does not join in. You have assessed her as competent to complete the physical task but she will need to be reminded that the patient is as much in need of human conversation and inclusion in the activity as she is in need of bathing. You evaluate the learning needs of the student as interactive communication with her patient. This then forms the basis of your next teaching activity.

Reflection

- Do the educational taxonomies, the teaching cycle and teaching plan help you to see this activity as teaching, learning and assessing as well as a care intervention?
- Should you tell the student during the bed bath that she needs to talk to the patient?
- How can you find out why she did not talk to the patient?

As can be seen above the teaching cycle does not end at the end of the individual teaching intervention covered by the teaching plan. At the end of this episode you can evaluate her needs for the next learning instance and use this to plan the next intervention, and so on. As the student progresses through her placement you will continuously assess her progress along with the other RNs on the placement. To make an accurate assessment of her learning you should take into account one of the hierarchies of learning to see how she is progressing.

These theories can be used in everyday practice and will enhance the experience of teaching, learning and assessing for the senior student or RN and for the learner.

How you will be assessed

All pre-registration courses will have an aspect of teaching and learning theory within them. You may be expected to provide evidence as part of a formal assessment. However, whether you are or not, your lecturers will be assessing your ability to understand the concepts above. If you can bring into your reflective writing and discussion that you have conducted an activity similar to the one described in Case study 5.1, your lecturers will see that you have understood and been able to apply the theory to practice.

Reflective learning

As well as being about to understand theories related to teaching, you should also be able to show you can engage in learning based on reflection. All nursing programmes have reflective practice built into them. This is because it is a central tenet of nursing and an indication of professional practice. One of the main indicators of a professional is that they constantly reflect upon their actions and try to improve upon them (Schon, 1991). You will have been taught a number of reflective models or cycles. You can help other learners to reflect upon their actions by the use of these and show your educators that you have done the same in your reflections.

References

Anderson, L. W., Krathwohl, D. R. and Bloom, B. S. (2001) *A Taxonomy for Learning, Teaching, and Assessing: A Revision of Bloom's Taxonomy of Educational Objectives*. Complete edn. New York and London: Longman.

Benner, P. (1982) From novice to expert, *The American Journal of Nursing*, 82(3): 402–407.

Benner, P. E. (1984) *From Novice to Expert: Excellence and Power in Clinical Nursing Practice*. Menlo Park, CA: Addison-Wesley Publishing Company, Nursing Division.

Biggs, J. (n.d.) *SOLO Taxonomy*. Available at: http://www.johnbiggs.com.au/academic/solo-taxonomy/ (accessed: 10 December 2015).

Biggs, J. B. and Tang, C. (2011) *Teaching for Quality Learning at University: What the Student Does*, 4th edn. Maidenhead: McGraw-Hill/Society for Research into Higher Education/Open University Press.

Bloom, B. S. (1956) *Taxonomy of Educational Objectives: The Classification of Educational Goals – Handbook I: Cognitive Domain*. New York: Longman.

Dave, R. H. (1970) Psychomotor levels, in Armstrong, R. J. (ed.) *Developing and Writing Behavioral Objectives*. Tucson, AZ: Educational Innovators Press.

Krathwohl, D. R., Bloom, B. S. and Masia, B. B. (1964) *Taxonomy of Educational Objectives: The Classification of Educational Goals: Handbook II: Affective Domain*. New York: Longman.

Nursing and Midwifery Council (NMC) (2008) *Standards to Support Learning and Assessment in Practice*. London: NMC.

Nursing and Midwifery Council (NMC) (2015) *The Code: Professional Standards of Practice and Behaviour for Nurses and Midwives*. London: NMC.

Schon, D. A. (1991) *The Reflective Practitioner: How Professionals Think in Action*. Aldershot: Avebury.

Whitehead, W. (2010) *An Investigation into the Effects of Clinical Facilitator Nurses on Medical Wards* [electronic resource]. Available at: http://etheses.nottingham.ac.uk/1264/

6 **Passing your assessments**

Overview

Learning is the main purpose of education and the point of the final year in the university setting is to provide nurses with the knowledge that they need to care for patients safely and effectively. However, all of this learning is of no use unless the examiners are satisfied that you have embedded the knowledge and are able to communicate this to the required standard. By this point in your programme you will have developed skills and strategies that suit you and help you to meet this standard. This chapter focuses on revising the main study skills techniques and developing new ones in order to step up to the level 6 requirements of this stage of learning.

The final hurdle

One may argue that by the time you reach the final year of your nursing programme, you have acquired all the fundamental skills required and have developed your knowledge base to a satisfactory or 'safe' standard. The task now is to assimilate all this information, knowledge and skill in order to manage your patient, yourself and a team effectively. You need to ensure you can problem-solve and use your diagnostic reasoning to determine the appropriate course of action and care required for the patients in your care.

For instance, is it life threatening? Should action be prompt? Is it ethically right to be treating this patient if he is confused and unable to give consent? There will be many more dilemmas to be dealt with and these will undoubtedly be challenging. However, you should remember that being able to assimilate what you have learned and apply it in practice is the reason you undertook all the education, practice and assessments. This is your challenge as you move forward, and it will have its high points but equally there may be some difficulties. Ultimately, it is the ability to reflect, make sense and gain further knowledge and understanding to enable you to learn from both the positive and not so positive events that will make you an excellent, safe, competent and compassionate registered nurse (RN).

The final year will help you gain confidence of your clinical and theoretical skills, ascertain any weaknesses and address them, and integrate your knowledge. You may have a 'light bulb' moment when suddenly things make sense. Some may feel this earlier than others so do not be alarmed if you still feel it is not coming together. The important thing is to keep positive and seek guidance from your lecturing team and clinical staff, such as mentors or supervisors, because they are there to help and guide you. On qualifying everyone wants to be a 'safe' and competent nurse with the necessary skills and knowledge to practise effectively and efficiently.

In all honesty, the learning curve when you start as a qualified nurse will be a steep one. You are not only getting to grips with your new role but you may also be in an unfamiliar healthcare setting, a speciality you have not experienced during your programme, as well as dealing with new people who you have not met before but who you have to work with cohesively – ensuring you are adopting a team approach for the benefit of all staff in the environment and, most of all, the patients and their loved ones. This may be called an 'orientation' and, although major and at times overwhelming, it is just that. Your nursing programme prepares you for that orientation by assessing your competency, knowledge and understanding. This is achieved in a practice and theoretical setting as you need to be proficient in both elements.

Case study 6.1: Laura

Laura is about to embark on her management placement (the final practice element within her nursing programme). She has passed all her theoretical work to an extremely high standard, which will have a significant impact on her final degree classification. She is thrilled but is extremely nervous about going into practice. She has been in the acute environment and has managed to avoid drug rounds as they scare her. She has avoided any delegation as she does not feel confident around others, so has managed to carry out tasks herself. Her mentors in her previous placement felt she that she had worked hard but were concerned about her ability to work at the required level. They feel it is a matter of confidence and so she passed her penultimate placement with the recommendation that she worked on this area and that she needed to ensure she undertakes a number of drug rounds on her last placement as they are an essential part of the qualified nurse role.

Reflection

- Is there a problem with Laura becoming a qualified nurse currently?
- If she is excellent academically, is this enough?
- What could Laura have done prior to this point in her nursing programme?
- What are your responsibilities as a student nurse regarding your learning?
- What can Laura do in her final placement to gain the required knowledge and understanding?

Laura appears to have avoided important aspects of her learning. The qualified nurse role does not only involve being knowledgeable; that is, having a good academic and theoretical understanding of the concepts and theories underpinning practice. It also involves being able to practise in a safe manner. Drug administration and understanding regarding medication administration is a vital part of the role and inability or lack of competency can lead to patient harm. In addition, lack of delegation skills can create dysfunctional team dynamics and if a qualified nurse tries to care for their patients in isolation, then some tasks may be unfinished, not be undertaken or performed to a poor standard due to lack of time. This will inevitably lead, once again, to patient harm. It is not too late for Laura. She needs to be clear with her mentor about her needs and ensure a proactive and detailed action plan is in place to allow her to develop the skills required, but also to help her gain the confidence needed to progress and complete the programme.

How and why are you assessed?

Academic assessment in the final year may be varied. Research and appraising research is a crucial part of the nursing programme and in your final year you are expected to integrate it fully within all your work. You may be asked to perform a written assessment; for example, a literature review, a systematic review or an examination of a case study where referencing and appraising the research evidence will be fundamental to the outcomes you propose. Your teamworking abilities may be evaluated by getting you to engage in team tasks. The reason for this is that the examiner needs to determine your understanding surrounding theory and practice, assess your criticality when faced with an issue or theory and assess your practice in certain situations through simulated activity; for example, an objective structured clinical examination (OSCE) or role play.

There are many ways an assessment of your knowledge or skills can be ascertained; the important fact is that they are needed so that you can be safe in the knowledge that you are competent and have a satisfactory understanding. It should reassure you that you can question theory and apply it to practice determining the impact it may have on the way you deliver care to that patient or number of patients but also the impact on that patient's well-being and quality of life.

Another reason for you being assessed is academic credibility. Academic credibility is important as a registered professional as one is expected to advance understanding in fields of practice, to contribute to improving care or the way treatment is delivered and this is achieved through research, appraisal of evidence and dissemination of knowledge (Gazza and Hunker, 2012).

The success in your academic writing is influenced by a number of issues, which can be described as intrinsic and extrinsic factors, challenges and 'enablers' (Gopee and Deane, 2013). You should have the intrinsic and extrinsic motivation to write as you are embarking on the final stages of your journey into the profession you have worked so hard to enter. As nurses progress through their programme of study, you may be faced with challenges, either personal or professional, that affect your motivation; for example, a failed assignment, an ill sibling, deterioration in your health. These may be overcome by drawing on many different resources including your own will, the help of loved ones, your peers or the institutional support available through lecturers, meeting with study support advisers or using well-being facilities.

As you draw closer to your transition to registration, you will be driven by motives such as wanting to achieve a high classification, wanting to work as a qualified nurse, to make a difference, to be autonomous or just to prove to yourself that you will be a good staff nurse. By this point the challenges to effective academic writing should hopefully be resolving themselves, and although not everyone can attain 100 per cent in their coursework, achieving as good a grade as you can should be rewarding. You will do this through accessing support to help to develop your writing style but also through reading, as this may also help to develop your own style. The 'enablers' mentioned earlier are things that can help you to achieve your goals. These can take on a great number of guises, from assessment feedback that allows you to feed-forward with your work, peer support, structured student support sessions that help you to address limitations in your academic style to tutorial support. These can make a huge difference therefore the advice is to access whatever is there. Avoiding writing for fear of failing is not an advisable route and results in a greater chance of failing, and as you sense this, it feeds your fear. Allowing greater time for planning and writing is more advisable, especially if you find you struggle with ideas and the ordering of those ideas.

Case study 6.2: Leah

Leah was conducting a literature review for her dissertation and it was her final theoretical module. She wanted to examine choices surrounding preferred place of care for those with life-limiting illness. She needed to pull the commonalities within the research findings by examining the participant's responses within the seven studies she had found. She found three dominant themes that she wanted to address through her discussion section. She looked at the methodologies and some had recruited from a very small area, which was a predominantly Catholic community. Some of the interviewers were the people caring for the participants while some were informal carers who were the participants. She began to describe the findings and report the methodologies used.

She went to see her tutor with a section of her discussion. The tutor read it and asked 'What difference does it make if the interviewers also happened to be the staff providing that care?' She replied that they may not be truthful fearing upsetting the interviewer. The tutor replied, 'Why not put that in then? It is a valid point and demonstrates that you have a greater understanding and a critical viewpoint surrounding how they have undertaken the research.' They then went on to discuss bias and the importance of using a research textbook to help support her appraisal of the methodologies employed.

The tutor then discussed the small group and asked what the issue was. Leah began to realize that to be able to demonstrate her understanding she would need to question the findings and suggest the limitations of them, and also that the findings need to be applied to the general population, considering, for example:

- Does having choice about preferred place of care apply to everyone?
- What if there were patient safety or carer safety issues? Have these issues been included in the research findings?
- From the participants, responses were there any common or frequent suggestions or preferences and if so how did she think that they could be facilitated in the healthcare provision currently available?

Leah began to understand that her opinions were important because they had been formed on the back of her experience, understanding and research, and therefore demonstrate her higher level of thinking. The tutor reminded her that she should take care however because her opinions were not fact, and to indicate this she could use phrases like 'perhaps . . .' or 'a possible solution may be . . .'

Keeping in mind the learning outcomes

Skills for writing effectively should have been developed during your programme of study. Whitehead (2002) has suggested that early in nursing programmes students should identify what is needed from them in terms of academic writing. They should understand how academic writing and scholarly activity influence their ability to care. As you are about to embark on your professional career, you will have developed this understanding and hopefully the skill of academic writing. Some manage to achieve this easily while other students require more help and support for extended periods. There are things you can do to try to improve your chances of success and attaining a good classification for your degree. Key points include checking that the learning outcomes have been considered and answered as these form the basis of your assessment. If you fail to address or answer a learning outcome adequately, then you may risk failing the assessment. If there is an assessment guide to how marks will be awarded, consider this. Descriptive text at level 6 warrants little or no marks. Descriptive text may introduce your discussion but it does not carry much academic skill or demonstrate your advanced understanding. An examination of a case study will require you to briefly outline the case but there is no skill in outlining it. The skill is in the analysis: how you introduce theory to the discussion and apply it to the case, how you consider that theory, are there issues or limitations when considering the case? How could this be improved?

The marking criteria should be based on those learning outcomes. Remember that you will need to address all the learning outcomes but some may require more discussion than others. You need to identify what the focus of the assessment is. The marking criteria will be based upon you achieving adequate address of those learning outcomes so always check and recheck them as your work progresses and, more importantly, before you submit your work.

Help! I need structure

There is a variety of texts and journal articles written to help you get the best out of your academic writing and to improve your skill. Wright (2010), Wright and Ferns (2010) and Wright et al. (2011) provided a series of articles to help with the fundamentals of writing, from 'how to structure your work' to 'how and why you should make sense of the literature' (as discussed in Case study 6.2). They make useful suggestions including how the flow of your work can be improved by ensuring there is a progression from one point to the next and that signposting within the script can improve your presentation significantly. Your ideas need to be presented clearly and logically. Great ideas that start but are not taken forward

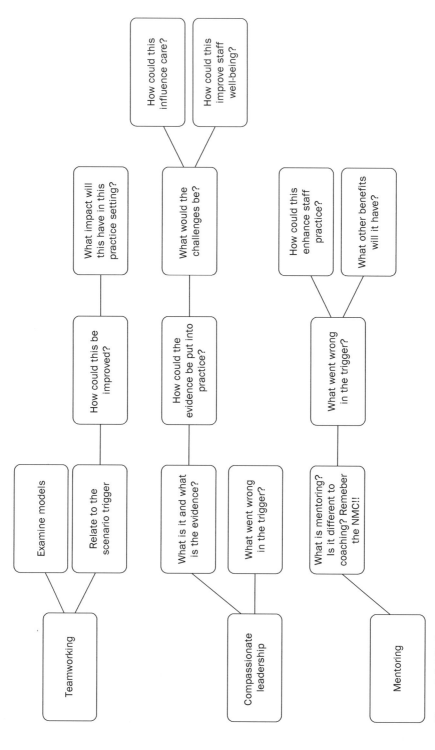

Figure 6.1 Mind map

or at worst lost in a sea of unclear unstructured sentences and paragraphs can seriously affect the final piece of work.

Generally, if a student has not planned a piece of work, it can be quite evident to the reader. The work often fails to progress logically. It feels like a surprise when a new aspect is mentioned, and it is as if you are trying to follow their thought processes but failing to do so. Logical progression means you take the reader through ideas and evidence in a reasonably obvious manner but the merit comes when you discuss that evidence in more depth before progressing to the next point. Issues should not be raised several times in slightly different ways, which is often the case without a plan – as you may have forgotten that you mentioned it earlier or you have had further inspiration so you mention something else relating to that issue or point. Planning allows you to cover necessary aspects, identify and consider the arguments and then move from A to B in a logical manner. Mind-mapping or just listing the content can all help with this.

Figure 6.1 is a mind map to help you to understand how they may help process your thoughts, facilitate deeper thinking and structure your work. These are not for everyone. You need to find what works for you. Consider a clinical situation where there was an absence of compassionate leadership, poor teamwork and lack of mentoring. The mind map grows as you ask more questions about those themes. Take a look and see if you can come up with more questions.

Pulling the discussion together

The other requirement for level 6 often involves identifying gaps in knowledge or limitations of evidence, suggesting new ideas or concepts utilizing those existing ones and addressing the contentious protestations made within the literature. You need to link theory to practice and this has been a consistent requirement throughout your programme of study. This can be seen as you will know already it is not enough to simply understand how the heart works, but it is also essential to understand how the heart might malfunction, and then to understand how this malfunction may be displayed in the care of the patient. From then, it is understanding what the evidence is to support and inform your care and, as important, if not more important, what impact does all this have on the patient and their well-being and how are you going to change practice and improve future care for people like this in your role as an RN?

And finally!

To demonstrate the higher level thinking, and to provide evidence that learning will continue to influence your practice, you will also need to make recommendations for future practice and applications. Identifying how this new understanding through the examination of theory and practice will improve your own practices; you need to say specifically how you are going to apply this. This demonstrates renewed understanding and acknowledgement that you can apply not only the theory but also your critical appraisal of the theory. You can then implement this into your practice to enhance the care you deliver.

References

Gazza, E. A. and Hunker, D. F. (2012) Facilitating scholarly writer development: the writing scaffold, *Nursing Forum*, 47(4): 278–285.

Gopee, N. and Deane, M. (2013) Strategies for successful academic writing: institutional and non-institutional support for students, *Nurse Education Today*, 33(12): 1624–1631.

Whitehead, D. (2002) The academic writing experiences of a group of student nurses: a phenomenological study, *Journal of Advanced Nursing*, 38(5): 498–506.

Wright, K. (2010) Simple writing skills for students, part one: structure and clarity, *British Journal of Nursing*, 19(11): 709–711.

Wright, K. and Ferns, T. (2010). Simple writing skills for students, part two: researching your subject, *British Journal of Nursing*, 19(17): 1118–1120.

Wright, K., Street, P. and Gousy, M. (2011) Academic skills: using literature to support your discussion, *British Journal of Nursing*, 20(2): 101–106.

PART 2

Practice (or how to perform well and to learn the skills needed as a final year student in practice preparing for transition to registered nurse)

7

How to prove to your mentor that you are fit to join the register

Overview

This chapter discusses what mentors and other registered nurses (RNs) want to see in the final year student. The main themes are confidence in your abilities and knowing your limitations. This chapter also covers issues such as when to be a team player and when to speak out effectively (see also Part 3).

Introduction

Ever since your first placement in the first year, you have been continually assessed by RNs. However, in your final year this becomes even more serious because the RNs on your placement are now assessing whether they can see you as a newly qualified nurse (NQN) working alongside them. On your final placement you will need to demonstrate that you are fit to join the register. Consequently, in your final year you need to demonstrate to your mentor and to other RNs that you are already able to function at the level of competency required of an NQN. This is a tricky thing to do because, of course, as a student you will not be permitted to do a range of the activities that an RN is allowed to do and you will continue to require the supervision of an RN. This chapter helps you to assess how best to approach your placements.

This chapter also acts as an introduction to the other topics that are covered in this second part of the textbook, and why these topics are important to your practice. It also concludes with consideration of when to report concerning issues on final year placements.

How to be confident in your abilities and to know your limitations

You are a senior student. Any conversations you have with more junior students will indicate how far you have come. It is worth either working alongside more junior students or seeking nursing-related conversations with them in order to judge your progress. Whether you can do this or not, you should be confident in the knowledge that by your final year you will have built up a bank of clinical skills from your experience on placement and in university.

Reflection

Find some of your assignments, reflections or revision writing from your first year. Read your work with third-year eyes. Some of it is likely to appear insightful and knowledgeable. Some of it is likely to read as naïve and simplistic.

- What do you learn from this?
- Do you still agree with your first-year self?

You may find that the placements you have experienced in the early stages of your course are similar to those in your final year. If that is the case, you will be able to use your experience directly and build upon it. However, many students reach their final year and land upon a placement that is very dissimilar to any they have had previously. This is very likely to happen in the modern nursing environment because nursing has become such a broad profession and placements have followed this trend. If you are in an area that appears totally alien, your experiences will be less obviously transferable. However, your previous placement exposure has made you capable of learning new skills more quickly.

The design of many programmes is around the hub and spoke model (Sherratt *et al.*, 2013). Hub placements are the main experience where the student's practice is assessed and are often up to a year in length. The spokes are short placements or simulated practice, designed to provide additional exposure to nursing specialisms, sometimes consisting of a few days (often known as 'insight visits') and no more than a few weeks.

This programme design has the advantage, as Roxburgh *et al.* (2012) found, of increasing depth of learning. Nevertheless, it often means that students remain on one placement for longer and consequently have fewer different experiences of clinical environments (see Case study 7.1 for an example of this).

Case study 7.1: Third-year placement

A student nurse is undertaking a three-year BSc (Hons) in nursing. He has completed his first two years and is now entering his first third-year placement on an acute medical ward. His placements have so far been with a community nursing team; a hospital operating department; a nursing home; and an outpatients' department. He has had some 'insight visits' to hospital inpatient areas but these will not have provided the depth of experience to give him that instant familiarity with the workplace that inspires confidence. However, during his previous placements he had experience of working with nursing and multidisciplinary teams (MDTs); providing fundamental care to patients; caring for unconscious and vulnerable patients; giving injections; following an aseptic technique for wound dressings; and using his nursing communication skills in complex situations while being involved in the holistic care of a wide variety of patients.

Reflection

Do a strengths, limitations, opportunities and challenges (SLOC) analysis as shown in Figure 7.1 that focuses on the student in Case study 7.1 as starts his first final year placement. In the top two boxes you will need to identify the strengths and limitations of the prior experience of this student. Then for the 'Opportunities' box, consider the opportunities in the forthcoming placement for the student to build upon the strengths gained and to mitigate the limitations of not being in a similar environment before. For the remaining box, consider the challenges created by this placement and reflect upon how the student can deal with these when entering his third-year placement.

- How can the student utilize the advantages and mitigate the disadvantages identified above?

From the SLOC analysis, build an action plan for him to take to the placement to ensure that the required activity and support is utilised to make the most of this experience.

Strengths	Limitations
(existing self-perceived personal strengths)	(self-perceived personal development needs)
Opportunities	Challenges
(available opportunities on placement)	(potential barriers to addressing personal development needs on placement and how they may be overcome)

Figure 7.1 Strengths, limitations, opportunities and challenges (SOC) analysis template

Your confidence in your abilities is best developed by a realistic appraisal of your existing skills, knowledge and experiences. This can provide a platform upon which to build your learning needs for the next step. Remember that you are still a student and your practice-based mentors will expect you to have learning needs as well as existing experience from the earlier stages of your programme. In fact, as you will see in the final section of the book, this learning journey will not end at the point of registration. It will carry on throughout your career as a nurse (Nursing and Midwifery Council (NMC), 2015b).

Brief overview of the rest of the chapters in this section

It is important to note that the whole of this section is about proving your ability to be a qualified nurse to your mentor, yourself, to colleagues and to your patients. When you read and interact with the following chapters, think about using the things that you learn to prove to RNs that you are ready to join the register (Bondy, 1983). These chapters are:

8. Thinking like a staff nurse
9. Practising like a staff nurse
10. Holistic care of the patient
11. Know your speciality
12. Leading a team on a hospital ward
13. Managing a caseload in the community
14. Effective delegation
15. Key skills of the staff nurse
16. Passing your sign-off mentor assessment
17. Applying for and obtaining your first registered nurse position

As you will see, consideration of each of these subjects will contribute to an overall impression of a practitioner who is fit for purpose, practice and award.

If you get into the mind-set of trying to think and practise like a staff nurse in your third year, then those around you will be able to visualize your competency as a newly qualified practitioner. This is important at the beginning of your final year as well as at its end because it is important to ensure that your mentor, as assessor, can envision your progress to this goal. Consequently, this should be your aim from day one of your third year. Advice on how to do this is outlined in Chapters 8 and 9.

The next two chapters on holistic care and knowing your speciality may sound like opposite ends of the spectrum. The first encompasses the whole of the individual: mind, body, spirit and social being, whereas the second is about the specific medical and nursing care focus of the placement upon which you find yourself. Nevertheless, these are not only mutually compatible ways of looking at individual patient care and the organization of caregiving; they are also important aspects of that knowledge set required by all professional nurses. The ability to look at holistic well-being, as well as speciality knowledge, is therefore crucial to convincing others of your worthiness to join the professional register.

The ability to lead a team in hospital (Chapter 12) and to manage a caseload in the community (Chapter 13) is essentially proving the same set of skills in the appropriate setting. One of the most important roles of the NQN is to be able to manage the competing needs of a group of patients. Whether this is in a community setting where each individual is visited in succession or in a hospital environment where the care can be provided in a closer geographical area is less important than the ability to prioritize and provide the correct interventions. The particular ways of doing this are different depending on the setting but the principle remains the same.

In order to provide care to a number of people effectively, the staff nurse often needs to delegate appropriate parts of their role (Chapter 14). This is one of the set of skills required by every nurse that novice nurses often find the most difficult both to learn and to implement. Again, the ability to do this effectively is an essential indication of your ability to provide competent care as an NQN. In the same way the senior student should ensure that they know the key set of skills expected of the NQN (Chapter 15). Delegation is clearly an important example of these skills. Nevertheless, of course, there are a set of skills in addition to delegation that need to be learned and enacted. Some of these are likely to have been mastered prior to the final year but others will need to either be enhanced or learned in the run up to qualification. Either way the final placement 'sign-off' mentor is likely to want to be sure that you have gained competency in the fundamental as well as the more advanced skills required of the nurse.

When you reach this final stage, the level of scrutiny of your practice is likely to be at its greatest because the assessing practitioner is aware that their decision will be the final hurdle to registration. Consequently, their assessment at this stage (Chapter 16) will permit or deny your entry to the register. This final 'performance' as a student will lead to your ability to work in your first position as an RN. However, it is likely that the interviews for this first job will be conducted prior to achieving registration. As a result, applying for and obtaining your first RN position (Chapter 17) is likely to take place during your final year as a student. The ability to take up this offer will be dependent on passing your final placement, therefore the effort put into these two activities needs to be carefully considered and appropriate weight given to both.

The ability to prove yourself to your mentor is dependent on your ability to demonstrate competency in all of the subjects covered in the chapters in this section. The central idea behind this is impressing upon your mentor that you have the skills, knowledge and experience to perform as a staff nurse at an acceptable standard. However, this does not just mean doing things to please your mentor. It is as important to be critical of existing practice as to be able to demonstrate your ability to perform as a team player in the workplace. Being a team player and speaking out against poor practice should not be in opposition to one another. However, the realities of healthcare workplace cultures can lead to these two activities being seen as mutually exclusive (Sawer and Donnelly, n.d.). As a professional this should not be a consideration you have to make, either morally or legally, as your duty as a nurse is for the well-being of your patients. This difficult position is now discussed.

When to be a team player and when to speak out

As alluded to above, one of the most important parts of being an RN is being a team player. However, there are times when going along with the majority opinion is not appropriate (Whitehead and Barker, 2010). The NMC has guidance on raising concerns (NMC, 2015a) and the issues related to being a new RN and this dilemma are covered in more depth in Chapters 18 'How to become a valuable part of the team' and 19 'When to speak out'. Nevertheless, there is a particular problem related to being a student that differs to those of being a new RN. It could be that as a student you are only a few weeks away from being qualified and so you may have a similar level of knowledge or skill to a new RN to base your judgements upon. The main difference, as a senior student, is that you are not yet on the register. Consequently, your mentor has the power to accept you into the profession or not. This means that you have a particular interest in maintaining a good relationship with that one person, which is much 'higher stakes' than any that you will have as a qualified nurse. Even your manager, as an RN, is not in such an influential position over your future career as your mentor. In addition, as an RN you have the professional autonomy to change jobs whenever you choose. This is one of the great attractions of the profession. However, as a student you have limited power to influence your allocated placement or mentor, for the most part. Should this make you comply with the realities of practice in order to achieve your goal of becoming an RN?

It is true that proving to your mentor that you are fit for the register is essential to becoming qualified. Nevertheless, this must be balanced against your duty as a future nurse to take action where you see wrongdoing. If you are found to have complied with an individual or culture which was not conducive to good care, that could also have a bearing on a mentor's decision to sign you off as ready for registration. In any case, it is both a moral and legal responsibility to take action even if that action leads to detrimental results for you personally at the time. The difficulty is that these dilemmas are unlikely to be related to clear-cut issues that obviously should be reported, because where they are someone will generally have beaten you to it. It will often be more nuanced cases where staff are not following the most current guidance or have to prioritize care due to staff or resource shortages outside of their control. These are hard and difficult decisions and the exercises in Chapters 18 and 19 are as pertinent to a senior student as to an RN to help you to work through this minefield. You should also seek advice from senior staff in the placement setting or in the workplace and in your university to help you through these decisions. The university staff are a resource that you have in order to support you in making these sorts of difficult decision and as a student you should make use of it while you remain a student.

References

Bondy, K. N (1983) Criterion-referenced definitions for rating scales in clinical evaluation, *Journal of Nursing Education*, 22(9): 376–382.

Nursing and Midwifery Council (NMC) (2015a) *Raising Concerns: Guidance for Nurses and Midwives*. London: NMC. Available at: https://www.nmc.org.uk/standards/guidance/raising-concerns-guidance-for-nurses-and-midwives

Nursing and Midwifery Counci (NMC) (2015b) *Revalidation*. London: NMC. Available at: https://www.nmc.org.uk/globalassets/sitedocuments/revalidation/how-to-revalidate-booklet.pdf

Roxburgh, M., Conlon, M. and Banks, D. (2012) Evaluating Hub and Spoke models of practice learning in Scotland, UK: a multiple case study approach, *Nurse Education Today*, 32(7): 782–789.

Sawer, P. and Donnelly, L. (n.d.) Meet the NHS whistle-blowers who exposed the truth, *The Telegraph*. Available at: http://www.telegraph.co.uk/news/health/news/11398148/The-NHS-whistle-blowers-who-spoke-out-for-patients.html

Sherratt, L., Whitehead, B., Young, A., Collins, G. and Brundrett, H. (2013) Using more healthcare areas for placements, *Nursing Times*, 109(25): 18–21.

Whitehead, B. and Barker, D. (2010) Does the risk of reprisal prevent nurses blowing the whistle on bad practice?, *Nursing Times*, 106(43): 12–15.

8 Thinking like a staff nurse

Overview

Schön and others have argued that what makes a professional is reflection in action. However, this is, as you may know, only part of the way you need to think as a staff nurse when you are on duty. The things that you need to know and understand as a staff nurse will develop as you practise. Your core needs are to ensure you are safe. In addition, considering the needs of your patients, colleagues and yourself is fundamental in everyday practice. You will develop as you begin to gain experience, confidence and competency. This chapter addresses some of the challenges but should also reassure you that many newly qualified nurses (NQNs) will have similar challenges and that these can be overcome.

Introduction

The Code dictates what we should and should not do within our practice (Nursing and Midwifery Council (NMC), 2015). This is about protecting our patients, relatives, colleagues and ourselves. Our practice will develop as we become more experienced and much of this lies in the ability to reflect on our learning. Reflection on action (Schon, 1991) is only part of what we do or think while on duty. As we move into the role of the NQN, there may be some anxiety as a student nurse surrounding the transition. Additionally, as the transition occurs, there may be some disparity between this perception and the reality, which again may induce some anxiety, or, alternatively, it may provide some relief if the perception was worse than the reality. As a student you have a mentor to ask, guide, teach and support you. Sometimes we can think that our responsibilities will change as soon as we start the role of staff nurse and we will be expected to deal with patients, relatives and other interprofessional colleagues to name but a few by ourselves. Although we definitely will have to deal with all these disciplines and professionals, and so on, we will not need to have all the answers to their questions on day one. One may argue that we may never have all the answers and this is a very positive thing as this motivates us to learn more.

As an NQN, the nature of preceptorship allows for this transition period so that we can learn and become familiar with thinking like a staff nurse. It is not some innate experience that occurs the night before we put on our first qualified nurse's uniform. One should be reassured that every nurse goes through this experience and each will develop in their own unique way. It resembles a rite of passage!

The patient

Obviously, it is the patient that drives our desire to be safe, effective, competent and efficient. We do not want to harm them through lack of knowledge, or to have them unsupported through poor time management, for example. We need to feel equipped to undertake the role well.

Thinking like a staff nurse may not happen overnight but takes experience, reflection and learning. What one needs to ask is, does thinking like a staff nurse come with being a staff nurse? How realistic is it to think that we can wake on that first morning and feel confident and have the ability to manage our team competently and effectively as if we were born with this innate skill? The answer is that this is unlikely. There may be instances where NQNs feel well prepared and unphased by their new role but it depends on where their job is, their previous experience and their own personality. For many students, what their programme of education has done is equipped them to be safe. This is not unique to nursing but may be similar for all those entering a health profession. In nursing, a safe practitioner is a good place to start. Furthermore, it has taken a number of years to complete your nursing programme. You have undertaken a number of assessments from a variety of staff in consultation with service users, other professionals, and your clinical practice has been scrutinized, therefore be reassured that all these experiences will have made you ready for the transition.

Case study 8.1: John

John finished the final day of his nursing programme. He felt he was ready for his staff nurse role. He had done really well in his last assessments and his final mentor was impressed with his clinical practice. He was due to start work on a busy surgical ward the following week.

His first day came and went in a profusion of uncertainty, feeling overwhelmed, unprepared and in awe of the staff nurses who appeared to competently carry out their roles. He began to question himself, his assessments and the length of his programme - had it been long enough to equip him with the knowledge and skill he needed to embark on this journey and role?

John is displaying perfectly reasonable feelings and raising questions that many NQNs and, perhaps, other healthcare professionals may ask themselves when embarking on the role they have worked hard for. Often we may have unrealistic expectations regarding what we would expect or should expect of ourselves. You are not underprepared; you are competent, but now need to build your confidence and specialist knowledge in the particular area of practice that you have embarked upon. It may be useful to discuss the writing of Benner (1984); although a dated text, its premise surrounding this paradigm still resonates today. Benner described being a novice and gradually, through experience and further professional development, there is a transition into the expert role within their area. This expertise does have some transferable elements but is not entirely transferable. When the expert moves into a different area or field of practice, they often regress through the levels of knowledge and cease to be the expert. This uncertainty and questioning his practice that John feels is part of that journey. He is no longer a true novice as he has transferable skills but also he has meaningful and essential knowledge gained from his programme of learning. This will develop over time and with that confidence will grow. He will use his experience gained as a staff nurse to further develop his competency and expertise but, if he changes role or area, once again he will experience some uncertainties and identify deficits in his knowledge, although this will not be quite as significant as his first day of his nursing programme or his first day as a staff nurse.

Competency

The qualities associated with being a good staff nurse may sound, to some, super-human and may cause one to question whether a person with all these qualities exists. Patients have expectations of the nurse caring for them that may lead us to question whether we could ever fulfil their needs, and in addition to this, our own expectations, and those of our colleagues, may feel a little daunting.

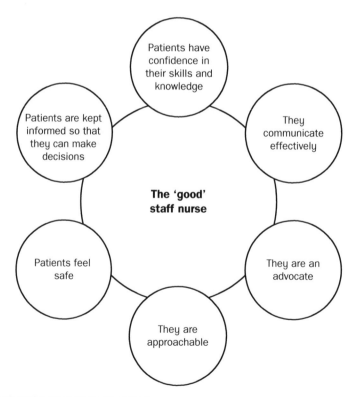

Figure 8.1 Patients' perceptions of nurses

Source: Adapted from Fradd (2010), cited by Ritchie (2013).

You do have many, if not all of the qualities, in Figure 8.1, and certainly having the competency and knowledge surrounding keeping a patient safe is also one of the prerequisites before transfer to registration can occur. The remaining qualities identified in Figure 8.1 may be present but at different levels and these will develop rapidly as you embark on your new role.

Worrying about how competent and safe you are may be a reasonable concern. Feeling competent surrounding not just fundamental care, but also care needs of critically ill patients, diagnostic reasoning skills, a broad understanding of a range of fundamental pharmacology, adequate understanding of anatomy and physiology, as well as understanding the disease trajectory of more common conditions can all help to ensure greater safety. It also increases one's ability in identifying risk and greater health and welfare issues for patients in your care. There is no doubt that caring with attributes like compassion (Brown, 2016) is vital, but so too are the areas of knowledge just listed, because this knowledge informs good care and compassionate practice. If you feel that you have weaknesses in knowledge surrounding core skills or issues, then whether you are about to register or have already registered, you need to ensure you attain this essential knowledge. The fact that you recognize it will be seen as a strength, it is not something to feel ashamed about.

Thinking like a staff nurse involves behaving like a staff nurse. The public and our colleagues may have expectations regarding a set of professional behaviours deemed 'appropriate' (some examples are listed in Fradd, 2010, cited by Ritchie, 2013), and a level of competency. Keeling and Templeman (2013) examined student nurses' perceptions of what it was to be a professional nurse. They identified that being a nurse means you are a nurse 24/7; in other words, you have to behave in an appropriately professional manner even when you are not at work. This perhaps is the concept that people have in the general population. This set of behaviours, or a way of being, may be encapsulated and referred to as 'professional behaviour' and includes qualities like being compassionate and courageous (NMC, 2015). Wynd (2003) identified that often other professions have basic descriptions surrounding sets of tasks associated with the specific profession, but in nursing, this has additional connotations that involve additional expectations; for example, behaviours appropriate to the nursing profession, autonomy, self-regulation, having a sense of vocation. One may argue that these expectations are quite simplistic, and that these may no longer be deemed 'essential'. In fact, these core values like having a sense of vocation, seem to be experiencing a revival in light of failures in the healthcare sector where professional behaviour appears to have been in question (Francis, 2013; Care Quality Commission (CQC), 2012). There are many arguments surrounding the influences and extrinsic issues impacting on a nurse's performance in these instances and many similar situations. Qualities and requisites of a nurse encompass the recognition that they need to be compassionate to others, have the ability to be empathic, to provide dignified care. These are not academic requirements but are just as important as a nurse's knowledge surrounding medication; for example, their diagnostic reasoning, their ability to link theory to practice, and their competency in managing a group of patients and their loved ones.

Case study 8.2: Joanne

Joanne is a third-year student nurse. She has struggled throughout her nursing programme to attain the academic standard required for her degree. In practice, however, she feels comfortable. She always goes the extra mile to ensure her patients feel cared for and listened to. Often she becomes engaged in difficult conversations that she then asks if she can share with her mentors to ensure they get the appropriate support and information they need. She engages with all her colleagues and provides a great deal of support to all who work with her. She tries to consider her patients' needs and to understand the issues and their concerns. Out of work, she is considerate and has never done anything to compromise her position.

In her interview for a staff nurse, she realizes that the other interviewee is one of the students on her university programme who has always achieved high standards in her work, and her knowledge base is excellent. Joanne becomes despondent because this is the job she really wanted as the patients, due to their situation and condition, would require a great deal of support. She felt that this was the type of nursing she loved.

She is overwhelmed when she discovers she got the job! Although she was thrilled, she was perplexed as to why her fellow student did not get it. When given feedback, they commended her on her enthusiasm and her very apparent compassion and desire to help make a difference to patients going through distressing experiences. The overall professionalism she displayed made her the ideal candidate.

Academic attainment and knowledge base is essential but it is not the only requirement of a staff nurse. Having sensitivity, self-awareness, enthusiasm and humility may be as important to ensure patients get the high standard of care they should receive. Joanne demonstrated this in her interview as she told of her experiences.

Being a staff nurse is not just about your knowledge; it is about how you use that knowledge for the benefit of your patients and colleagues. It was in 1986 that the United Kingdom Central Council (UKCC) for Nursing (2000) launched the revolutionary Project 2000 nursing programme and stated that what was needed for the future was a nurse who was a 'knowledgeable doer'. As a staff nurse, you may want to be more than just a knowledgeable doer. You may want to think about:

- What impact that knowledge can have on your practice?
- Are there any deficits?
- What are the alternatives?
- How could you do it better?
- What do you need to develop it further?
- How you can deliver care encompassing compassion, dignity and empathy that is needed to provide a high standard of care

As a staff nurse you need to think about your practice, reflect on action and in action to be able to answer these questions. It may be helpful for you to consider your role as a whole and identify your strengths, your weaknesses, the opportunities it offers and challenges that may lie ahead (see Figure 7.1 for a useful way to lay out this type of analysis).

You are not born a nurse and you do not reach the end of your nursing programme an expert. Nursing is a lifelong journey of discovery involving human interaction which, at times, may be distressing or joyous, challenging or confusing, and yet all these experiences can help to shape you, as a nurse, in order to help you care with insight for others, but also to share your insight with others.

Case study 8.1 (*continued*): John

John was described in Case study 8.1. He completed his first week as a nurse, then his first month, and then his first year. He managed to complete his preceptorship and go on to be a mentor. He was commended for his teaching skills, his care, and his compassion to patients and his colleagues. He recognized that nursing is exactly what he needed to do and to do it with the level of care that ensured patient comfort. Sharing this with others was something he felt passionate about and he wanted to inspire others to do the same.

References

Benner, P. E. (1984) *From Novice to Expert: Excellence and Power in Clinical Nursing Practice.* Menlo Park, CA: Addison-Wesley Publishing Company, Nursing Division.

Brown, M. (2016) *Palliative Care for Nursing and Healthcare.* London: Sage.

Care Quality Commission (CQC) (2012) *Our Role in Winterbourne View: Internal Management Review.* Available at: http://www.cqc.org.uk/sites/default/files/documents/20120730_wv_imr_final_report.pdf (accessed: 2 September 2016).

Fradd, E. (2010) *Gradually Graduating to Graduateness: The Impact of Nursing Becoming a Graduate Profession.* Conference paper presented at the University of Nottingham, 20 July, cited by Ritchie, D. (2013) The professional nurse: image and values in nursing, in Hall, C. and Ritchie, D. *What is Nursing? Exploring Theory and Practice*, 3rd edn. Exeter: Learning Matters.

Francis, R. (2013) *The Mid-Staffordshire NHS Foundation Trust Inquiry Report.* London: The Stationery Office.

Keeling, J. and Templeman, J. (2013) An exploratory study: student nurses' perceptions of professionalism, *Nurse Education in Practice*, 13(1): 18–22.

Nursing and Midwifery Council (NMC) (2015) *The Code.* London: NMC.

Schon, D. (1991) *The Reflective Practitioner: How Professionals Think in Action.* London: Ashgate.

United Kingdom Central Council (UKCC) for Nursing, Midwifery and Health Visiting (1986) *Project 2000.* London: UKCC.

Wynd, C. A. (2003) Current factors contributing to professionalism in nursing, *Journal of Professional Nursing*, 19(5): 251–261.

Practising as a staff nurse

Overview

Staff nurses need to use a range of skills and knowledge to function effectively. These are learned during their pre-registration education and in experience and continuing professional development (CPD) following registration. When asked what is the most important skill in nursing the usual response from registered nurses (RNs) is 'communication'. In addition to communication, the RN needs to have an air of confidence in the way they show their competency levels, as well as the competency itself to carry out the work. In this chapter ways to conduct yourself and show skills in these areas and others are explored and examined.

Introduction

The contents of the preceding chapter and this one are intrinsically linked and intertwined. However, the result of thinking like a staff nurse is appropriate action, and it is the combination of thinking and action that leads to the activities in the clinical area that we think of as nursing practice. That is not to say that everyone agrees that the sole point of thinking for a nurse is the activity which results. As Drennan and Hyde (2009) argue, the need for study to lead directly to improved practice is sometimes disputed by academics in nurse education. The right balance here must be sought. The pursuit of learning for its own sake is a laudable activity, but, as a professional discipline, the main reason for studying and for expanding understanding through research is to improve practice. This is the case as an individual practitioner as well as a standard for the profession. This is what the idea of the 'knowledgeable doer' (Drennan and Hyde, 2009) encapsulates.

Considering your level of skill and knowledge

Nurse education is designed to produce an RN who can make a start in any nursing environment as an NQN. In your first job after you qualify, you will be expected to become knowledgeable and skilled in that specific area of practice. Consequently, when you are on placement as a final year student it will be expected that you quickly come to grips with the placement's specific clinical and caring focus. It may be that you have not had practical experience in a similar area to the one you will experience as a senior student. This often leads students to feel anxious about their ability to function at the higher level of competency expected at the final stage of their programme (Bondy, 1983). However, if you consider the things that you need to know and do in order to practise like a staff nurse, then this should not be a problem. This is illustrated in Case study 9.1 and Reflection that follows.

Case study 9.1: Dawn

In the first two stages of her course, Dawn had placement experiences in a hospital theatre; a district nursing team; a hospital outpatients' department; and a nursing home. In her final year she was placed onto a busy hospital medical ward. Her mentor, Eve, sighed when she heard this and said 'Why don't they prepare students for their third year anymore? We'll have to teach you from scratch'.

Dawn has had a perfectly respectable range of nursing experiences as they are all possible working environments of the RN and they include patient experiences in the community, the hospital and the home. The skills and knowledge that this will have provided Dawn in preparation for her experience as a third year on a medical ward include:

- fundamental care skills
- airway management
- IVI maintenance
- care of the unconscious patient
- manual handling
- communication skills with the multidisciplinary team (MDT)
- communication with patients
- knowledge of the requirements of patients on discharge from hospital to their own home and to a nursing home
- medication administration
- many other nursing skills appropriate to this clinical area.

In addition, Dawn will have learned, and been assessed on, a range of pertinent topics in university. These will often include clinical simulation activities covering many of the above skills and even simulated ward situations. The classroom, online and library-based university learning activities will have included reflective practice, healthcare ethics, anatomy and physiology, psychology, sociology and government policy. All of these are important preparatory learning for the final year placement in whatever area.

Consequently, the experience that Dawn's mentor is seeing as lacking is experience of the hospital ward environment rather than the nursing skills that she will need in order to function in that environment. When entering any unfamiliar clinical environment it is necessary to have plenty of guidance and support to 'learn the ropes'. Nevertheless, not having experienced care on a hospital ward should not be a problem if you take the skills and knowledge accumulated in the first stages of the programme and apply them to this new environment.

It will be necessary for Dawn to familiarize herself with the ward routine and speciality but she will not need to be treated like a first-year student.

Reflection

The mentor is clearly incorrect in believing that she will have to start from the beginning in preparing Dawn to function at the level required of a final year placement.

- If you were in Dawn's place, how would you respond to her concerns in the scenario?

Communication skills

As indicated above, communication skills are among the most important abilities required by nurses. The key skills of the staff nurse are covered in more detail in a later chapter but it is worth considering the communication skills needed to show that you are practising like a staff nurse here. These are important skills for clinical practice and as a student. In your clinical practice you are interacting with patients, their family and friends, and the MDT. In your student role you are communicating with other students, placement mentors and university lecturers. In the first two years of your course, communication skills will have been part of the curriculum. In addition, you will have experienced examples of good and bad communication styles in your placements and personal life. The theory and practice of communication methods will have prepared you for the more demanding communication requirements of the senior student nurse on placement.

There are many theoretical frameworks for communication beyond the basic understanding that for communication you need a *sender*, a *message* and a *receiver* (McQuail and Windahl, 2013) and that much of the meaning is purveyed in tone of voice and facial expression (Mehrabian, 1971). Most of the more recent models are based on empirical evidence and therefore can be confirmed by observation. One of the most widely known and used is transactional analysis (Berne, 1961). In Berne's transactional analysis model, the sender or receiver of the message can take on the role of parent, adult or child (see Figure 9.1). If neither party in the communication exchange is aware of their or the correspondent's role, this can lead to misrepresentation or misunderstanding of the intended meaning on either part.

These theoretical frameworks can help us communicate in the real world as they provide enhanced ways of interpreting the message that we may not pick up intuitively simply from life experience. An example of miscommunication is indicated in the case study which follows.

Case study 9.2: Dawn and Eve

Student nurse Dawn's perspective

Dawn has been on the medical ward placement for three weeks. Her mentor, Eve, has been asking her lots of questions about the care for patients in her team and the routine of the ward. Some of these have appeared to Dawn to be critical of her practice as Eve has been asking her '*Why* are you doing that?' to everything she does. Towards the end of the shift Eve asks Dawn if she has seen her stethoscope anywhere. Dawn replies to Eve, 'Why do you always blame me for everything?'

RN Eve's perspective

Eve is working with her mentee Dawn. She has spent a lot of time teaching Dawn the ropes over the last few weeks and she is pleased to see that Dawn has quickly picked up the ward routine and understanding of the medical conditions and treatments. She has decided to find out the extent of Dawn's learning this week in order to make sure that she is prepared to take charge of her patient care next week. Consequently, she has been asking questions to ensure that Dawn understands, as well as being able to carry out, the clinical tasks required. She is really pleased with the majority of her answers and feels ready to let her try leading the team, under supervision, tomorrow. Dawn realizes just before it is time to go home that she has misplaced her stethoscope. She is just about to retrace her steps to look for it and asks Dawn if she has seen it. Eve is surprised to see that Dawn becomes upset and accuses her of blaming her for everything.

If we use the ideas of communication related above to pick this apart, we can see that there is a misunderstanding between the two parties in the conversation throughout the day. Eve had intended to put across a positive message that her student was doing well and almost ready to progress to the next stage in her practical assessment. Dawn perceived that her mentor was being critical and finally believed that she was blaming her for things going wrong. Using the transactional analysis model this appears to be a parent to child discussion from Dawn's perspective and an adult to adult conversation from Eve's perspective. This is what Berne describes as a crossed transaction (Berne, 1961) and this is illustrated in Figure 9.1.

AGENT			RESPONDENT
Parent			Parent
Adult			Adult
Child			Child

Figure 9.1 Crossed transaction communication in Berne's transactional analysis

Case study 9.2 illustrates a situation where unintended messages are passed both ways. This could probably have been avoided by the mentor explaining at the outset the purpose of the exercise and by her praising the good work that she thinks that Dawn has been doing.

Reflection

- Can you recall any similar discussions?
- How could you use communication theory to improve your ability to practise like a staff nurse?

How to be seen as confident and competent

Entering a new or a familiar environment as a third-year student is a daunting experience. Your mentor will be expecting to see you perform at the level of the staff nurse that you will become once you have made the transition from student to RN. Consequently, they will expect you to perform your duties in a confident and competent way. This means that you must not only *be* proficient in your practice but you must *be seen to* be proficient. Our recent systematic review indicated that the perception that NQNs are not competent is in error (Whitehead *et al.*, 2012; Whitehead *et al.*, 2013). It seems that competency is not the problem. NQNs, on the whole, have the broad range of skills required for entry to the profession. It seems to be that there are two issues for NQNs and therefore for final year students trying to show that they are fit for the register:

1. The first issue is that nursing is a very wide profession and includes work in many patient care environments. Consequently, students have been prepared for any nursing post, in any clinical arena, rather than for this specific position, therefore they cannot have the specialist skills and knowledge for the place that they are allocated for their final year placement or for their first job. They will need to 'learn the ropes' to acclimatize to the routines and policies in whatever workplace that they find themselves and they will need to gain or update knowledge in the conditions and treatments most common in that area.
2. NQNs appear to have the required skills to commence their careers safely. 'Forneris and Peden-McAlpine (2009), Holland *et al.* (2010), Fox *et al.* (2005) all found that, to a certain extent, NQNs and their managers were less confident in the NQNs' ability to perform tasks competently than objective measurements showed them to be' (Whitehead *et al.*, 2012: 34). What they don't have is sufficient confidence in their ability to perform these skills. Consequently, they may appear to others to be lacking in ability due to their hesitancy to demonstrate their ability.

As a final year student, aiming to show to your mentor that you are able to perform at the required level; therefore, it will be necessary to make sure that you either have, or can gain, the knowledge and skills specific to the placement area and to be able to demonstrate at every opportunity to your mentor and others that you have acquired them. This is likely to mean reading up on the most frequently encountered medical conditions for the placement area and practising as soon as possible the main roles of the staff nurse, such as drug administration, liaison with the MDT and managing a team. If these experiences are not offered to you by your mentor you should ask for them, as otherwise you may not get the opportunity to practise until you are the only one available to do it, possibly after you have qualified.

Case study 9.1 (*continued*): Dawn

Dawn has been on her placement for seven weeks. She is well liked by the healthcare assistants (HCAs) and RNs as she is always ready to 'muck in' with feeding, washing and toileting patients who are unable to perform these fundamental 'activities of living' due to their illness. Her mentor Eve has observed her progress and feels that she is now ready to be in charge of a bay of four patients for the day under her, arm's length, supervision. Dawn feels very uncomfortable about this as she does not think that she has sufficient experience to do it and certainly does not want to tell HCAs what to do.

Having a senior student lead a team, under the supervision of her mentor, is of course essential preparation for being an RN. Unfortunately, Eve has not prepared her student for this ahead of time and consequently Dawn does not feel confident in her ability to do it even though her mentor has assessed her as ready. Eve could have prepared Dawn for this experience by having her shadow her mentor or another RN with a view to doing this on a specified day. This would have indicated to Dawn and her mentor that she was fully prepared for the day. It is easy for students to fall into the routine of providing general care alongside non-registered staff. It is often the role of carer that attracted the learner nurse to study for the profession. The roles that only the RN can perform, such as delegation of caring duties to HCAs, drug administration and liaising with other professionals appear less attractive. They will also, rightly, have spent a great deal of time and effort in perfecting these caring skills, as they are a central part of the RN role. However, the senior student now needs to take these nursing foundations and build their more advanced skills onto them.

Reflection

Eve felt that Dawn was ready to use her knowledge of the ward to practise the role of the staff nurse under her supervision and assessment. Dawn did not agree with her mentor's assessment of her ability. Clearly, in Eve's opinion Dawn had the competency.

- How could Dawn have improved her confidence to fulfil her mentor's expectations?

Conclusion

The final year student needs to show her mentor and the other staff on her placement that she has the skills, knowledge and confidence to perform her duties as an RN, otherwise her mentor will assess her abilities as not being sufficient to join the register. In order to do this, she needs to practise like a staff nurse. This does not mean simply copying the behaviours of her mentor although, so long as the student sees her as a justified role model, then this should be part of the strategy. It means that the final year student should use her existing knowledge and experience to inform her practice and to both think and act like the nurse that she wishes to become. This could sound like arrogance as she has not yet joined the register. However, if she cannot visibly demonstrate the confidence and competency she will need, then it will be difficult for her mentor to assess her ability to be a nurse.

References

Berne, E. (1961) *Transactional Analysis in Psychotherapy: A Systematic Individual and Social Psychiatry.* New York: Grove Press; London: Evergreen Books.

Bondy, K. N. (1983) Criterion-referenced definitions for rating scales in clinical evaluation, *Journal of Nursing Education*, 22(9): 376–382.

Drennan, J. and Hyde, A. (2009) The fragmented discourse of the 'knowledgeable doer': nursing academics' and nurse managers' perspectives on a master's education for nurses, *Advances in Health Sciences Education*, 14(2): 173–186.

Forneris, S. and Peden-McAlpine, C. (2009) Creating context for critical thinking in practice: the role of the preceptor, *Journal of Advanced Nursing*, 65(8): 1715–1724.

Fox, R., Henderson, A. and Malko-Nyhan, K. (2005) They survive despite the organizational culture, not because of it: a longitudinal study of new staff perceptions of what constitutes support during the transition to an acute tertiary facility, *International Journal of Nursing Practice*, 11(5): 193–199.

Holland, K., Roxburgh, M., Johnson, M., Topping, K., Watson, R., Lauder, W. and Porter, M. (2010) Fitness for practice in nursing and midwifery education in Scotland, United Kingdom, *Journal of Clinical Nursing*, 19(3/4): 461–469.

Mcquail, D. A. and Windahl, S. A. (2013) *Communication Models for the Study of Mass Communications*, 2nd Edn. London: Routledge.

Mehrabian, A. (1971) *Silent Messages.* Belmont, CA: Wadsworth.

Whitehead, B., Holmes, D., Beddingham, E., Henshaw, L., Owen, P., Simmons, M. and Walker, C. (2012) *Preceptorship Programmes in the UK: A Systematic Literature Review* [online]. Available at: https://docs.google.com/file/d/0Bzzvt7Tfz8TKZEhNSkl5bmtyelk/edit?usp=sharing (accessed: 6 May 2016).

Whitehead, B., Owen, P., Holmes, D., Beddingham, E., Simmons, M., Henshaw, L., Barton, M. and Walker, C. (2013) Supporting newly qualified nurses in the UK: a systematic literature review, *Nurse Education Today*, 33(4): 370–377.

10 | Holistic care of the patient

Overview

In your final year you will be expected to be able to provide patient-centred care. In the previous years you will have learned the various components of care and by this stage you should be able to put these together to provide fully rounded care. Consequently, this chapter deals with providing holistic care for the patient.

Introduction

As a healthcare professional you have significant responsibility regarding the safety of your patient. This safety requires methodical assessment, robust, responsive planning and the delivery of competent, safe, effective and compassionate care. This should all be achieved using a holistic approach. Holistic care does not only mean ensuring the patient's physical needs are addressed but equally important are their social, psychological, spiritual and emotional needs (Brown and Hardy, 2016). The Department of Health (DH) (2008, 2009) identified further requirements of holistic care and suggested that environmental, financial and cultural aspects should be addressed in addition.

Your pre-registration nursing programme will demand competency in the thorough and robust assessment of your patient. As a staff nurse your responsibility and accountability to ensure this is achieved is undeniable (Nursing and Midwifery Council (NMC), 2015).

Assessments are not only undertaken in a hospital environment. As health and social care becomes more diverse, the areas where assessments may be required will consequently be more diverse, ranging from a variety of private, voluntary and independent institutions to the more traditional areas like a patient's home or an acute hospital ward. Wherever they are undertaken, however, health and social care professionals need to maintain the same comprehensive holistic philosophy and the intention should be that the patient is as involved in their care as much as possible (Howatson Jones *et al.*, 2012).

The patient-centred approach

Holistic assessment and care delivery is not undertaken in isolation. It involves working with other professionals and non-professionals in order to deliver seamless, responsive care that corresponds with patient wishes and requirements. This suggests that the patient is key to the decision making, which is the crucial issue. Patient empowerment in the assessment and planning process should be fundamental, as without patient involvement, we cannot identify what they want, what they need and what their goals are for the future. Issues that we may consider a significant burden to them may not be a burden for the patient. We have to use our communication skills to not only advise, but, more importantly and more crucial in this partnership, to also listen. Enhancing your listening skills in the communication process can aid therapeutic engagement between the patient and health and social care professional (Payne *et al.*, 2008). This can engender a rewarding therapeutic relationship promoting trust. The principle of 'no decision about me without me' (DH, 2012: 13) emphasizes the importance of collaboration in this holistic care partnership in order to achieve the compassionate care we wish to attain.

Case study 10.1: Neil

Neil, a 42-year-old, with ulcerative colitis, was admitted for a bowel resection to the inpatient surgical unit. He smokes 15 cigarettes per day, has a wife and two children aged 7 and 9. He is a self-employed plumber. His BMI indicates he is mildly obese.

The nurse admits him to the unit for surgery the following day. He has already commenced his bowel preparation and is in some pain. The nurse needs to get on with his admission as there are five other admissions awaiting assessment. She goes through the activities of daily living and acknowledges he cares for himself, eats regularly, has no special diet, and his bowels are frequent with episodes of urgency and bleeding hence his resection. He has had courses of steroids with little effect. His religion is Church of England and in terms of his sexuality he lives with his wife and children. She talks him through the surgery explaining about pre-medication which may be given but mainly about his return to the ward. As health promotion is a nurse's responsibility she quickly advises him that he should try to stop smoking and lose a little weight. She offers the smoking cessation service for this and he accepts.

Reflection

- Consider how the nurse deals with this patient admission. Do you think this could have been achieved using a more holistic approach?
- If you do, what aspects do you think are missing?
- How do you think Neil is feeling?
- Could we do any more to address his needs?

Often we may find ourselves in stressful situations where it seems overwhelming and the only way to get through the day is to prioritize and cut corners while ensuring we remain safe and our patients are safe. Unfortunately, for people like Neil, it may mean that we leave patients feeling vulnerable and anxious, which is not a situation they should be facing alone. Both Barrett *et al.* (2009) and McCormack and McCance (2010) signified that this is a failure in care as patient needs are not met. If we assess Neil using a holistic approach, we may find other intrinsic and extrinsic issues, as Case study 10.1 (continued below) illustrates.

Case study 10.1 (*continued*): Neil

Neil has felt extremely unwell as his colitis has been poorly controlled with his medication. He knew that this was coming but, as he works for himself, he tried to avoid it as he was concerned about loss of income. He had decided to take a job working away from home as it would pay well but the distress of leaving his wife and children was almost unbearable and then, one month ago, his father died suddenly after receiving a diagnosis of bowel cancer only eight weeks before. He had not smoked for 20 years but as he was working away, he felt he needed a cigarette. His diet had deteriorated as he was living in a guest house and working so late that all he could manage to get to eat was takeaway food.

He is extremely anxious that the surgeons will find 'something else' when they operate. He is fearful for his wife and children as he does not feel he has provided enough for them should anything happen to him. In addition, if he does make it through the operation, he needs to get back to work as soon as possible.

Reflection

- Consider the issues raised by Neil's situation. Do you think we need to address these issues?
- Do you think they would have been captured in the admission by the nurse during her admission process?
- How can a holistic assessment identify and address these issues?

The nurse's responsibility

To leave a patient in a distressed state such as this through an inadequate assessment – that is, one that fails to incorporate a holistic approach – does not comply with our responsibility and accountability to the NMC standard 3 (NMC, 2015). We are duty bound to relieve suffering, to treat people with dignity and to ensure their needs are addressed. As a staff nurse you may not be able to meet all these needs and will undoubtedly require referrals to people like a social worker for financial advice, or getting the consultant to speak to the patient regarding (for example) his concerns about the potential for underlying malignant disease, as well as seeking out someone who is able to listen to him regarding his recent bereavement – note though that this could be you depending on how competent you feel. In this situation you would need to remember that grief is a normal process and he will still be grieving. He may just need to talk about his father's decline and try to make sense of it.

One cannot often separate physical illness from psychological well-being. Emotional distress may be evident in a patient who is suffering with ill health. It would make sense that to treat a person as a whole, you will have to assess that person as a whole, and care for that person as a whole, not seeing them merely as a set of symptoms or an illness label.

You should utilize robust strategies to facilitate a comprehensive assessment if required and then carefully structured and planned care can be discussed alongside the patient and potentially their relatives or carers if appropriate. The planned care that would be identified through a nurse's deeper conversation with Neil could be in a number of areas, as already indicated. If he receives information surrounding his concerns about malignancy, and if his anxieties surrounding his financial situation are addressed, he may feel in greater control of his whole situation. The therapeutic relationship that may evolve from this encounter may be rewarding for the professional involved but also invaluable to Neil.

The importance of communication

Communication is vital during this process. To create a safe environment where the patient feels they can share their fears and anxieties as well as their symptoms can ensure the patient receives the support and care they require.

Patients need to understand what your aims are when caring for them. Often they may identify their concerns and their symptoms from a biomedical approach as their perceptions are focused on physical illness and physical symptoms, while their anxieties and emotional distress, social issues, spiritual issues are considered 'their problem' rather than something to share with health and social care professionals. In Neil's case, he felt that his financial worries were his problem to sort out, yet they may have a significant impact on his recovery and may force him to return to work earlier than perhaps he should due to his worries about income (Pederson and Emmers-Sommer, 2012). Pederson and Emmers-Sommer (2012) undertook a qualitative study examining understanding surrounding their assessment and care. Ten participants were recruited. All had advanced, life-limiting disease so one may assume that their care needs may be complex with mortality concerns and emotional, psychological and spiritual distress being significant. In the study they had limited understanding surrounding how their holistic needs were being met and only focused on physical care when recalling what it was that they received from healthcare staff.

This perhaps demonstrates that we need to improve our communication strategies and make it clear what we mean by caring for the whole person and be specific with our patient surrounding the holistic philosophy. Although this is only one study, the fact that the World Health Organization (WHO) (2014) identified it as an international issue appears to concur with Pederson and Emmers-Sommer's (2012) findings. In this particular publication, WHO are referring to end-of-life care but one may argue that everyone with a health condition should be treated the same and have the same rights to holistic care. Without this philosophy, distress and poorly managed symptoms could ensue and without considering the whole person, care will undoubtedly be suboptimal, which is not what we strive to achieve.

It is quite possible that if the healthcare professional was to stress that the aim was to not only meet their physical needs but also to address all of the domains associated with holism, this may promote a feeling of safety and reassurance that they are being heard. It may also provide the patient with a perceived permission to discuss any issues that are concerning them rather than only those that they feel are of relevance, which, judging by the latter research study, are predominantly physical concerns.

Assessment tools

There are a variety of assessment tools that are designed to aid you in the assessment of your patient, including the Malnutrition Universal Screening Tool (Malnutrition Advisory Group, 2008) and the Modified Early Warning System (National Institute for Health and Care Excellence (NICE), 2007). Many of them are very specific and can help form part of the holistic assessment but there are also very generic holistic assessment tools available; for example, Roper *et al.* (2000). What can help you in the assessment and care planning is an understanding surrounding the presenting illness or condition, the evidence underpinning the care of the individual with the specific condition but also being prepared to learn from the patient about how it feels to have the condition, how it affects their lives and being able to consider other issues that may have an impact on their ability to live with the illness or condition.

Conclusion

You have a responsibility professionally, ethically and morally to provide holistic care. This includes the assessment and collaboration using a patient-centred approach in order to plan the care that meets the patient's specific, individual needs. Patients need to understand what a holistic approach is in order to engage in the assessment process because if they do not, they may fail to inform you or share with you issues relevant to their care and to care planning. Effective communication during the assessment and care planning process can, in itself, facilitate a therapeutic engagement and relationship between the health and social care professional and patient.

Compassionate care means wanting to understand suffering, and a desire to relieve that suffering (Brown and Hardy, 2016). To be able to do this, we all need to carry out comprehensive holistic assessments.

References

Barrett, D., Wilson, B. and Woodlands, A. (2009) *Care Planning: A Guide for Nurses*. Harlow: Pearson Education.

Brown, M. and Hardy, K. (2016) Holistic assessment, in Brown, M. (ed.) *Palliative Care in Nursing and Healthcare*. London: Sage.

Department of Health (DH) (2008) *End of Life Care Strategy: Promoting High Quality Care for All Adults at the End of Life*. London: Her Majesty's Stationery Office (HMSO).

Department of Health (DH) (2009) *End of Life Care Strategy: Quality Markers and Measures for End of Life Care*. London: Her Majesty's Stationery Office (HMSO).

Department of Health (DH) (2012) *Liberating the NHS: No Decision About Me Without Me*. London: Her Majesty's Stationery Office (HMSO). Available at: https://consultations.dh.gov. uk/choice/choice-future-proposals/supporting_documents/Choice%20consultation%20%20 No%20decison%20about%20me%20without%20me.pdf

Howatson-Jones, L., Standing, M. and Roberts, S. (2012) *Patient Assessment and Care Planning in Nursing*. London: Sage.

Malnutrition Advisory Group (2008) *Malnutrition Universal Screening Tool*. Redditch: Bapen.

McCormack, B. and McCance, Y. (2010) *The Theory and Practice of Patient-Centredness in Nursing*. Oxford: Wiley-Blackwell.

National Institute for Health and Care Excellence (NICE) (2007) *Acutely Ill Patients in Hospital*. Clinical Guideline No. 50. London: NICE.

Nursing and Midwifery Council (NMC) (2015) *The Code*. London: NMC.

Payne, S., Seymour, J. and Ingleton, I. (2008) *Palliative Care Nursing Principles and Evidence for Practice*, 2nd edn. Maidenhead: Open University Press.

Pederson, S. N. and Emmers-Sommer, T. M. (2012) 'I'm not trying to be cured, so there's not much he can do for me': hospice patients constructions of hospice holistic care approach in a biomedical culture, *Death Studies*, 36(5): 419–446.

Roper, N., Logan, W. and Tierney, A. (2000) *The Roper-Logan-Tierney Model of Nursing: Based on Activities of Living*. London: Churchill Livingstone.

World Health Organization (WHO) (2014) *Global Atlas on Palliative Care and End of Life*. Geneva: WHO. Available at: www.thewpca.org/resources/global-atlas-on-end-of-life-care (accessed: 24 May 2016)

11 | **Know your speciality**

Overview

This chapter discusses strategies to ensure you find out what you need to know about the placement speciality you are going to be allocated to. Methods of learning and retaining information about the clinical speciality and the practical care procedures are suggested.

What are the expectations?

It is your responsibility to know the area of practice you are embarking on and that you have examined the evidence that underpins the care to be delivered in the specific area of health provision to which you are allocated.

There are a number of facets to ensure that you fulfil the requirements or expectations of the placement. One is that you are expected to demonstrate a particular level of competency and this level rises as you progress through your programme, from a very basic level, whereby much of your time and care is very directed and supervised, to the point of transition to registration, where a level of responsibility is placed upon you. At this point you are expected to manage a caseload of patients as you will be required to do this as a newly qualified nurse (NQN). In addition to managing this caseload, you will have to demonstrate effective leadership, delegation, assessment and evaluation that are essential to ensure the safety of those in your care and to confirm to your mentor that you are a safe and effective practitioner.

In order to demonstrate you know your speciality, having an evidence-based understanding is fundamental. It is important to consider how you will develop your learning so that you do have an evidence base for how you act in your speciality.

Learning does not only happen in the classroom. Placements can provide a springboard for you to find out more and to help to identify limitations in your knowledge and understanding. It is imperative that you identify these limitations and try to address them through literature, guidance and the use of multimedia. For instance, interactive programmes for anatomy and physiology can be effective to ascertain the function of organs and systems, which may appeal to some rather than trying to understand it in a textbook.

Case study 11.1: Elsa

Elsa was on her management placement with a pulmonary rehabilitation team. She had undergone her induction and initial interview. The mentor had given her a variety of resources in order to help her achieve the requirements and competencies for the placement. In addition, she offered Elsa help and guidance as Elsa identified aspects she felt were unclear or difficult to understand. Elsa got to her third week and was asked if she wanted to lead a discussion for a patient who had been discharged following an exacerbation of his chronic obstructive pulmonary disease (COPD). Elsa felt anxious but agreed as she had witnessed these discussions a number of times since starting the placement. Elsa started to describe the condition and identify what the intended treatment outcome was. The patient then began to ask questions and Elsa found she could answer them accurately but also in a way that the patient and his carer understood. The mentor did not need to step in and was really impressed with Elsa's knowledge and understanding as well as her commitment to her learning.

At the end of the day the mentor and Elsa sat down to discuss the consultation. It became apparent that Elsa had read beyond the background reading identified by the mentor. She disclosed that anatomy and physiology was a weakness of hers but she was really interested in the patient's condition and this helped her learning.

Reflection

What were Elsa's responsibilities to

- herself?
- her mentor?
- her patient?

If Elsa had not been proactive in her learning or failed to acknowledge her weakness, the consultation with the patient would have been very different. Elsa demonstrated her desire to practise in a competent and safe manner; she could have endangered the patient if she had given out inaccurate information. If you are aware about any weakness in your understanding or practice, you, as an adult learner and a professional, have a responsibility to address it and seek guidance. Being responsible for your own learning is essential for safe practice and, with this, the acknowledgement of your limitations is important (Nursing and Midwifery Council (NMC), 2015). This does not mean that you should not try to address the limitations; on the contrary, you have the responsibility to identify learning opportunities to enhance your practice.

Many placement areas have resources that may help to determine what you need to know about caring for patients and relatives in that particular area. Some may be very specific (coronary care unit) while others may be quite broad (district nursing service). The resources have been developed to help you but also identify what the mentors feel is important for you to understand and learn. They are also more likely to give you time and opportunity to use them in your normal shift time rather than in your own time that may be limited due to other academic commitments. You must remember however that your learning is equally important in the clinical environment.

Having a discussion with your mentor can also help to identify where support for learning may be needed. Elsa discussed her difficulties with her mentor and they developed an action plan to address Elsa's difficulties. If you are aware of learning needs, then identifying them and addressing them through further study at this point as a student is vital rather than when you are a staff nurse. This would allow you more confidence in your practice and could ensure greater safety in managing future patients. As a staff nurse you would be expected to have a baseline understanding and then to develop your knowledge in the specific field of practice. Elsa should enlist further help from the academic environment to ensure that she obtains all the support available.

What is key, once again, and fundamental to this topic, is the recognition and the responsibility for your own learning and that learning should be at a deeper level than it was in your first year. So, rather than just learning about the heart or how to calculate drug dosages or how to complete an assessment, you should be aiming to identify the impact the illness may have on the individual, recognize when they may be deteriorating, understanding the care pathways and use your diagnostic reasoning skills in order to care for them competently. Although your skills will continue to develop when you are a staff nurse, trying to achieve a level of competency in areas you are allocated to can be of great benefit for your confidence and for the patient you are caring for.

Before the placement

Preparation prior to arriving at the placement can be a very effective way of learning and getting the most out of your placement. Reading about the speciality or looking for a website that they may have developed with information about it can help to identify what your priorities are for preparing for the environment. Being prepared and demonstrating you have done some preparatory work will work in your favour too as it will demonstrate to your mentor that you are enthusiastic and keen to learn. If you are interested in learning, you mentor may be more interested in teaching you. It is difficult, as a mentor, to maintain interest in someone who is disinterested.

Methods of learning

There are a number of ways you can learn and these can start before you enter your placement as already suggested. The benefits are that it helps you to link theory to practice as what you have read prior to entering the clinical environment may be something you can now witness. This can allow you to make sense of an illness or condition that you encounter and it may also help you to problem solve and question the situation. Following your initial investigation surrounding the speciality, examining specific cases may be an effective way to gather a more holistic understanding of the illness or condition.

Communicating with patients is a fundamental learning activity that can be underestimated. It is through patient narratives that a real depth of understanding can be generated. The lived experience of patients is crucial in order to respond in a compassionate manner to their suffering. Sitting down to listen to their experience of illness may help you to understand more about the condition than a physiology textbook may be able to tell you. It is often the living with it that defines how people cope and how it affects their life. This learning is crucial for you as a student nurse but more importantly as a staff nurse being able to respond appropriately to patients with specific conditions. Understanding the incidence of a condition, presentation and the signs and symptoms is important, but it does not tell us what worries the patients with those conditions or what it is like to live with the condition. This can only come through discussion, whether it be through communication between the nurse, patient and or relative/carer or through the undertaking of qualitative research.

Retaining information is about giving the information meaning and this often involves applying it. Reflection is an activity all nurses should be involved in. The NMC introduced revalidation for nurses in 2016, whereby nurses are required to reflect on their practice (NMC, 2015, 2017). This is not a one-off reflection, it should be done continuously. The revalidation process involves you producing a number of reflective pieces which identify your learning and allow you to link your knowledge, understanding and practice to the Code (NMC, 2017). Reflection is not a new concept and has been integral to a number of disciplines for years, but the NMC have determined that this should be a compulsory activity and should be documented. In addition, there is a responsibility to discuss the reflective activity with a professional on the NMC register in order to facilitate further learning (NMC, 2017). Being able to reflect on your experiences is therefore advocated, not just in your pre-registration programme, but also into your professional career.

Case study 11.2: Nigel

Nigel was undertaking his management placement in the community and was allocated to a team of community nurses. He was doing a dual visit with his mentor to a patient who had recently been diagnosed with advanced breast cancer. When they went to the house, her husband answered the door and he ushered them in. He looked pale and distressed. He explained that his wife was behaving oddly and was refusing to take any medication. The nurse asked Nigel to assess the lady and determine the plan of care. Nigel could not determine what the issues were as the lady was quite confused. She appeared distressed and in some discomfort. Nigel felt that they should give her some pain relief as she seemed to be suffering. When Nigel suggested an injection the lady refused, accusing him of trying to kill her. The district nurse stepped in and suggested that they contact the GP and get him to come and assess the lady as a matter of urgency.

Once outside the house Nigel was upset and felt he had left a patient suffering. The district nurse reassured him and discussed the issues surrounding the patient's capacity to consent. She suggested that Nigel may wish to reflect on this situation in order to develop his understanding but also to address his emotional distress at the situation. Nigel researched the condition but also went beyond this and examined the Mental Capacity Act (Parliament, 2005). He developed an understanding regarding some of the possible complications in advanced breast cancer that may have been attributable to the patient's confusion, and he also had a greater understanding surrounding consent and the procedures to be followed to protect those who do not have the ability to give consent, whether it be temporary or permanent.

Reflection

- Do you think Nigel will retain this learning? If so, why?
- How do you think the district nurse helped Nigel?
- Was it important for Nigel to go and search for information and evidence?
- Could the district nurse have saved him some time and sat and told him the information? Would this have been as effective?

As identified at the start of this chapter, a nurse has the responsibility for their own learning and Nigel is a good example here, because by seeking out the information that is needed to support his practice, he has engaged in what one may argue is a very 'real' and applied way of learning. Learning about a case study or a patient you are caring for may allow a greater understanding regarding how a certain side effect or complication can affect the patient. There may also be more motivation to learn where you have a real patient to care for too. Searching for information may be more effective than simply being told, as this is the underpinning philosophy of problem-based learning; it relies on the learner's own motivation and allows a more adult and pedagogical approach. In this approach, instead of the teachers identifying what the learning needs are, it is the learner who identifies their own learning needs.

Conclusion

Competency in a speciality relies on knowledge and attaining that knowledge can be achieved in a number of ways. Learners have individual learning styles and it is your responsibility to identify what works for you. What is undoubtedly crucial is that you recognize your need for knowledge, your weaknesses in your understanding and what support is available for you in order to meet your specific needs. Some core activities that should be carried out by nurses to help them recognize their learning needs and develop their knowledge are engaging in reflection and exploring evidence-based practice (EBP). Both of these involve an examination of current literature including policies, guidance, research and expert opinion. Once you have gained an understanding, it will help you to problem solve and, more importantly, care for your patients in a safe manner demonstrating a competent, knowledgeable approach.

References

Nursing and Midwifery Council (NMC) (2015) *The Code: Professional Standards of Practice and Behaviour for Nurses and Midwives*. London: NMC.

Nursing and Midwifery Council (NMC) (2017) *Revalidation*. London: NMC. Available at: http://revalidation.nmc.org.uk/ (accessed: 26 May 2017).

Parliament (2005) *Mental Capacity Act 2005* (chapter 9). London: The Stationery Office. Available at: www.legislation.gov.uk/ukpga/2005/9/contents

12 | Leading a team on a hospital ward

Overview

In Part 1 of this book, management and leadership theory were introduced. This chapter and the following chapter advises you how to put this theory into practice in your final placements. This chapter focuses on the skills needed to manage the care of a group of patients in hospital and together with the following chapter (13) also includes ways of working with a multidisciplinary team (MDT) in an inter-professional and collegiate manner best suited to providing the best patient care.

Introduction

One of the most important skills that the senior student needs to demonstrate in order to be assessed as worthy of joining the register is the ability to lead a team of nurses and carers to be able to provide holistic care to a group of patients. This is because the newly qualified nurse (NQN) starting work on a hospital ward will have this responsibility as the main part of their role. This chapter provides advice on the theory and practice of leading a team on the ward.

How to put management and leadership theory into practice

In Chapter 4 we provided an overview of management and leadership theory in nursing but this will not be returned to now. This section deals with putting the theoretical frameworks into practice. One of the biggest ideas in this field is that management and leadership are linked but different concepts. As Bennis (1989) determined, leaders 'do the right thing' and managers 'do things right'. Bennis listed attributes of managers and leaders to illustrate. However, the main point is that leaders take action to achieve the objective without too much concern about the existing rules; whereas managers ensure that the rules are followed without too much concern about the outcome. When you are leading a hospital ward team then both attributes of manager and leader are required of course. These attributes are in line with the grand theories of logical ethics; that is, deontology and utilitarianism (Whitehead, 2015). In ethical scholarship as well as in leadership theory these concepts are often seen as being contradictory. Much time and effort has been put into arguing for one or the other to be seen as the correct view of the world and hence the best way to make decisions and put them into action. However, in this chapter it is argued that the underpinning concepts in leadership theory, attributed to both 'leadership and' 'management'; and in ethical theory to both 'utilitarianism' and 'deontology', have merit. They are all theoretical frameworks worth considering when putting theory into practice.

In the section below, some thought experiments are provided as examples to illustrate the theories. These are not intended as advice on how to deal with the issues raised but are intended to be thought provoking. There are no easy answers in ethical theory and some of the discussions may be uncomfortable to read and it is likely that you will disagree with some of the actions described. However, that is the nature of the subject and the pages of a book are as safe a place to enter this difficult arena as any.

Ethical management

The moral imperative of 'doing things right' follows Kant's teaching on deontological ethics (Pojman and Vaughn, 2011); that is, managers and leaders should always try to make decisions based on the rules, professional guidelines or policies and procedure. On the whole this is obviously the right thing to do. The rules have been constructed in order to help people to make the right decisions. However, the absolute following of the rules implies that the person should never consider what will happen if they follow them but should only consider their duty to follow the rules no matter what the consequences are. Is this a reasonable way to live a good life as both a professional and a leader? Anyone who attempted to live their life this way would be an unusual person.

If we look at simple rules such as 'do not lie', it is easy to see the problem. Most people would agree that this is a sensible rule but the whole of peaceful society relies on everyone bending or breaking this rule every day in order to ensure that a good outcome ensues. In extreme circumstances only the most ardent deontologist would stick to the rule. For example, no one's life is perfect but each day when people ask 'how are you?' we often respond with 'I'm fine, how are you?' There are few people whose lives are entirely fine. On balance, yes, hopefully they are more fine than not, but the question was, 'how are you?', which demands some detail and a full answer would include a list of your aches, pains, concerns and minor as well as major difficulties. As can be seen from this benign example, it would make life very complicated if we all told the absolute truth all of the time. It could be argued that this is too simple a rule and that we need a number of exceptions or caveats. For example, we could have the rule to deal with the example above: 'only lie if you don't have time for the full answer and you think the person asking is just being polite anyway'. That would probably work for the example given but there are other reasons why the right thing to do is not tell the truth.

We could add to this rule to deal with other potential problems with absolute truth telling that we 'do not lie unless telling the absolute truth would upset someone'. This seems sensible but sometimes it may be right to upset someone in certain circumstances. In any case, this rule would be, by its nature, accepting that the consequence of an action, in this case 'upsetting someone', should lead to a different course of action. It is extremely difficult to devise a rule that considers every possible outcome in every situation where the rule may be applied. As a result, professionals have to make decisions based on their knowledge and experience as well as following the guidelines provided for them. That trust to make decisions is the privilege and burden of being a professional. Professional and workplace rules are usually more specific than the examples given above, but the same sort of problems can ensue. On the other hand, the deontological approach of 'doing things right' can often be a good way to support difficult decisions (e.g. see Case study 12.1).

Case study 12.1: Surgical placement

You are a senior student on your final placement on a surgical ward. You are preparing a patient who is just about to go to hand theatre and notice that they have a marker pen arrow on their right hand pointing to their thumb. You are sure that it was handed over that this person was to have surgery on their left thumb. You stop the porter and go to check the notes but the staff nurse asks why you are interfering with the process and states that you will delay the operating theatre list. You explain your concern but she says that this is unlikely and that they will double-check when the patient reaches theatre anyway. However, you know that the evidence-based World Health Organization (WHO) (2009) Surgical Safety Checklist Guidance and the National Patient Safety Agency (NPSA) (2010) Five Steps to Safer Surgery indicate that the marked site of surgery is one of the most common errors and that any member of the team should be empowered to speak up about concerns at any stage in the process. Consequently, you insist on checking the medical notes and show that your concern was correct. The error is avoided due to following the checklist rules.

A consideration of deontological management

This all sounds like the right way to go about your work as a professional and the Nursing and Midwifery Council (NMC) would certainly be in favour of registrants following the rules. However, there are a number of issues with the deontological approach to management:

1. Where do the rules come from? Is it evidence-based advice or just something that has always been done that way?
2. What happens when there is no rule for the specific situation that you are faced with?
3. If following the rule will lead to a bad consequence should you still follow the rule even though you know there is a better way?

Ethical leadership

'Doing the right thing' implies that the leader will assess their actions based on the consequences of their endeavours. This is in line with the thinking of utilitarian ethicists such as Bentham and Mill (Pojman and Vaughn, 2011). This implies that the leader should not consider what the rules are when making decisions but should try to work out what the action with the best consequence is. Of course, in the majority of cases, well thought-out rules will instruct the professional to take actions that coincide with the best outcome, as seen in Case study 12.1. The example of 'not lying' given in the previous section illustrates one reason why the consequence may sometimes be more important than the rule. In the case of lying or not lying, for most people it depends on the purpose, level and consequences of telling the truth or lying. As a nurse you should always be as honest and transparent with your patients as practicable but the everyday social niceties of not telling the absolute truth to every rhetorical question is common sense as well as ethically acceptable. Another example is when bad rules are made and the professional is obliged to break them. An example of this is given in Case study 12.2.

Case study 12.1 (*continued*): Surgical placement

You arrive, first thing on Saturday morning, to your placement on the surgical ward. The minimum number of registered nurses (RNs) that are required for the safety of patients on the ward is four nurses. However, you notice that there are only two staff nurses and the sister on duty. You mention this to your mentor and she tells you that the matron implemented a rule last week that if there was a senior student on duty at the weekend and that if an RN rang in sick they would not make any attempt to replace them. You complain to the sister that this means you are not considered to be supernumerary (NMC, 2010). She repeats the rule made by the matron and explains that a fourth staff nurse was on the rota to work but has rung in sick. You now have a dilemma as there are two rules that contradict each other. You consider the consequences of following the NMC rule or the matron's rule and you decide that the best course of action is to complete the shift and to discuss this with your university link lecturer on Monday. This decision is based on the projected consequence that patient care would suffer in the short term if you refused to provide care as a non-supernumerary worker. However, you are also considering the longer-term consequence of the matron's rule; that is, you and other students would not be supernumerary under certain circumstances that may have an adverse effect on your learning to become a competent RN (Shepherd and Uren, 2014). The university lecturer thanked you for bringing this to her attention and contacted the matron to explain that this was not an acceptable rule. The rule was withdrawn and supernumerary status for student nurses re-implemented on the ward.

A consideration of utilitarian leadership

Making decisions based on projected consequences of your actions is often seen as a more advanced skill than following the rules. However, it is not always the best route to follow. There are a number of issues with this utilitarian approach to leadership:

1. What if the outcome that you expected does not follow from the action you have taken?
2. If all leaders approach decision making in this way there are likely to be different judgements made with varying degrees of success. The logical

approach to this would be to assess the actions based on the consequences and devise an evidence-based rule that all leaders and managers should follow in similar circumstances.

3. Rules are probably best adhered to slavishly in emergency circumstances such as cardiac arrest: where very quick decisions need to be made and multiple scenarios have been carefully examined for the best evidence-based outcomes.

Reflection

1. Consider the second point in the list. Does this mean that we should always try to find an evidence-based rule, rather than trying to work out the best outcome for ourselves?
2. Consider the final point in the list. Are there circumstances, even in an emergency situation, where you should challenge the orthodox position?

Skills needed to manage the care of a group of patients in hospital

One of the most important skills in leading a group of nurses and healthcare assistants (HCAs) is making the best decisions. This has been covered at length above. In a hospital ward, once those decisions on what to do for the best care of your patients have been made, it is almost always necessary to delegate some of the care to a team. Delegation is covered in more detail in Chapter 14. This skill requires communication skills and leadership skills combined. If the team know that your guidance for making good decisions is often good they are more likely to follow your lead. This is especially the case if you use the communication skills covered in Chapter 9. In addition to gaining communication and leadership skills, leading a team requires the senior student to have built up knowledge of the common conditions and routine of the ward. The leader will need to know the individual needs of the patients in their care. Ideally, the leader will also know the professional interests and capabilities of the members of their team to ensure that they are directing them to the most appropriate work. All of this is complex but it is achievable when it is considered as a set of skills and knowledge to be learned and practised like any other professional responsibility. However, leading a team is often seen by nurses as the most onerous thing they have to do. This is especially the case for the student nurse practising this skill under the supervision of their mentor. Probably the largest obstacle to the student as leader is that most of the staff that they are learning to lead will be more experienced than they are. This challenge is illustrated in Case study 12.2.

Case study 12.2: Management placement

Your mentor feels that you are ready to lead the team for the section of the ward that you have been working in for the past few weeks. She says that she will be one of your team members for the day and that you must supervise the care of the patients. There is a first-year student nurse and two HCAs in the team to provide care for six patients. Usually, the staff nurse discusses the care of the patients and goes through what will be required for preparation for theatre, discharge and wound care for the day. However, today both HCAs just say that they know what they are doing and set off to start helping patients to get washed and dressed.

Reflection

- Why do you think that the HCAs have changed their routine today?
- What action should you take?
- Could you or your mentor have made this more successful by preparing the staff for your day of practising being 'in charge'?

Working with the MDT

Being in charge of the team does not of course end with those directly caring for the patients with you. There is a much wider MDT involved in the holistic care of the patients in your care. As the nurse in charge of your group of patients' care in the hospital ward, you are at the centre of this holistic care in the role of responsible, direct carer and patient advocate.

The inpatient experience in a hospital can be bewildering as the complex nature of modern healthcare requires a large number of specialized professionals to administer the best overall care. The MDT consists of professionals such as physiotherapists; occupational therapists; social workers; discharge co-ordinators; speech and language therapists; radiographers; chiropodists; psychologists; physicians of various kinds; a variety of specialist and generalist nurses; and many others. It is crucial for the nurse to know the roles and responsibilities of all of the professionals involved in the care of your patients.

The single, 24-hour-a-day constant is the ward nurses. For the nurse in charge this requires a high level of knowledge and communication. First, if this is you, you will need knowledge of the patients, their medical conditions and their social circumstances in order to ensure a safe discharge. Second, you require an all-round understanding of the roles of the MDT professionals as related to their patients' care. This is outlined below.

Case study 12.3 (*continued*): Management placement

The consultant surgeon has asked to conduct a ward round with your patients. She indicates that three of the patients have completed their surgical treatment and that they should be sent home. You are aware that one of your patients, Mrs James, was living alone in her house prior to admission but is now too weak to care for herself and needs two nurses to help her to transfer from bed to chair. The other two patients appear to be self-caring. You inform the physicians and the consultant notes this in the medical record and carries on with the ward round.

Reflection

- Which members of the MDT will you need to ensure are aware of the needs of Mrs James?
- Are the other two patients ready to be discharged home? How can you make sure?
- Is it the nurse in charge's responsibility to ensure the safe discharge of Mrs James and the other two patients or is it the consultant surgeon's?

Conclusion

Leading a team on a hospital ward is a complex role. It is also often considered to be a role that many student nurses and even RNs would rather avoid. However, it is important and necessary. It requires a set of skills and knowledge that can be learned rather than someone being a 'born leader'. If you take the time to learn the tricks of the trade it can be a rewarding role and if done properly will make the patients' journey through the ward a comfortable and effective one. Surely, this is the aim of all nurses?

References

National Patient Safety Agency (NPSA) (2010) *Five Steps to Safer Surgery*. Available at: http://www.nrls.npsa.nhs.uk/resources/collections/10-for-2010/five-steps-to-safer-surgery/?entryid45=92901 (accessed: 5 August 2016).

Bennis, W. G. (1989) *On Becoming a Leader*. New York: Addison-Wesley.

Nursing and Midwifery Council (NMC) (2010) *Standards for Pre-registration Nursing Education*. London: NMC.

Pojman, L. P. and Vaughn, L. (2011) *The Moral Life: An Introductory Reader in Ethics and Literature*, 4th edn. New York: Oxford: Oxford University Press.

Shepherd, P. and Uren, C. (2014) Protecting students' supernumerary status, *Nursing Times*, 110(20): 18–20.

Whitehead, B. (2015) *Deontology and Utilitarianism*. Available at: https://youtu.be/haI_s4zPgE8 (accessed: 21 July 2016).

World Health Organization (WHO) (2009) *WHO Surgical Safety Checklist*. Available at: http://www.nrls.npsa.nhs.uk/resources/?entryid45=59860 (accessed: 5 August 2016).

13 | Managing a caseload in the community

> **Overview**
>
> This chapter takes a similar approach to the previous one but looks at leading the care of a series of patients in a primary care setting. By the end of the chapter you will have the opportunity to examine the management and leadership theories introduced in the previous chapters related to practice in the community. You will then be encouraged to reflect on the interaction between you as the nurse and the rest of the multidisciplinary team (MDT).

Introduction

The final placement for a student nurse can be in any setting where registered nurses (RNs) work. Nevertheless, the majority of students will have their final placement either on a hospital ward or in a community nursing team. The previous chapter dealt with this stage on the hospital ward. There are many areas of similarity in the preparation for the experience of community nursing. The main thing that the mentor will be considering when assessing you in both arenas is whether you will be able to safely care for the group of patients in your care. Consequently, this chapter provides advice on the theory and practice of managing a caseload in the community.

How to put management and leadership theory into practice

The concept of ethical management and leadership in decision making has been introduced in the previous chapter. This is of similar value in managing a caseload in the community. In a community team you are more likely to be set the objective of managing a caseload rather than a community team because this is the level of responsibility usually experienced by the newly qualified nurse (NQN) starting work in a community team. The group of patients to be cared for are in their own homes rather than in a hospital ward. This presents an additional challenge as the nurse needs to prioritize and organize the care routine without being able to physically see each patient when planning the day's activities. This makes knowledge of the patients' conditions, psychological and social circumstances of at least equal importance to that needed on the hospital ward. The caseload of patients to care for is likely to be agreed in discussion with your mentor. They are likely to have taken you around their area for the first stage of the placement in order to ensure that you have met some of the regular patients and know where the base is and general layout of the area. This may mean that patients' homes are fairly close together if it is in an urban area or quite far apart if a rural community. The travelling time will need to be taken into account when planning the day. This is especially important when administering time critical medication such as insulin.

Management of a caseload of patients in the community requires good self-organization skills rather than delegation at the level that you are likely to be working. This can be a worrying responsibility as you may not have been given the responsibility of seeing patients alone to this extent before. Your mentor will be available in the same way as if you were on another placement and they will expect you to call them if you are in any doubt. Remember that the care of the patients remains their responsibility, as it does in any setting, while you are practising your ability to practise like a staff nurse.

Case study 13.1: Community placement

You are a senior student on your final placement on a rural community placement. You have agreed your day's workload of a group of patients with your mentor. The majority are patients with a variety of conditions that you have cared for many times during your placement. However, your third patient, Mr MacDonald, is a new client who has just been discharged from hospital following a chest infection that left him unable to care for himself for a period of time. The communication from the hospital indicates that he had a physiotherapy and occupational therapy (OT) assessment prior to discharge and that he was assessed as self-caring. Consequently, you are expecting this to be a routine check of a self-caring elderly man. However, on arrival you find that although Mr MacDonald can walk to the door to let you in he has struggled to do so and he tells you that he has not had the energy to make himself a cup of tea or anything to eat since he was discharged yesterday. You ring your mentor and she thanks you for raising this and asks you to stay with Mr MacDonald until she is able to come to see him herself.

Reflection

1. Why has this happened? Is anyone at fault?
2. If you were in this situation and knew that the next patient you were down to see needed their medication at a specific time how would you deal with it?
3. Has the student in the scenario used any specific management theory to make the decision to call her mentor? Was she right to do so as a senior student?

Working with the MDT

In Case study 13.1, the MDT had been involved in the discharge plan for Mr MacDonald. Nevertheless, he had not had a good transition from hospital to community. This could have been down to an error by the therapists and nurses assessing his needs. However, it is more likely to be that he had appeared well enough in the simulated experiences of home assessed in the hospital but had found the reality of coping at home more problematic. That is why the hospital team had asked the community nurses to check on him post-discharge. Similarly to the hospital setting, the care of patients is split between a large number of specialist practitioners. The list from the previous chapter can be added to with community matrons, district nurses, community mental health nurses, and many others. As it is with the hospital team, it is important to get to know the roles and responsibilities of the professions involved in your patients' holistic care.

Case study 13.1 (*continued*): Community placement

Mr MacDonald has managed to stay out of hospital as he has been assessed by his GP, the community matron and his care manager from the adult social services team. He has been assessed as needing a daily visit from a carer to help him to wash and dress himself and to assist him to prepare a meal. The community nursing team have been asked to maintain a weekly visit to assess his pressure areas as you had assessed him as at risk of pressure ulceration during your initial assessment (National Institute for Health and Care Excellence (NICE), 2014).

Your caseload includes patients needing insulin injections, wound dressings, hospital discharge assessment and nutrition assessments. You ask your mentor about the legality of administering insulin as a student. Your mentor explains that you are not in these cases administering the medication but are assisting the patient to self-administer. The drug is prescribed using a 'patient specific direction' rather than a 'patient group direction' (PGD) and, consequently, it is not necessary to be an RN to administer it. It is worth noting that if it were a PGD it would be illegal for a student or any other non-registrant to administer it even under direct supervision (Her Majesty's Stationery Office (HMSO), 2012) *The Human Medicines Regulations 2012: Schedule 16 Patient Group Directions*). At times, you are struggling to complete all of the care needed in the day before your official finish time. You discuss this with your mentor and she says that you are doing well but that the care takes longer when you first start and that you will become more efficient as you get used to it. She offers to help out with your caseload if necessary.

Reflection

- Which members of the MDT will you need to ensure are aware of the needs of Mr MacDonald and the other patients in your caseload?
- Do you agree with the mentor in this scenario that, with experience, you will become better at managing your time caring for a group of patients? Does that mean that as a senior student you should stay late in order to complete the workload agreed? Are there any risks involved in this?
- If the caseload includes drug administration, such as insulin injections, should you be doing this as a student nurse?

Conclusion

Managing a caseload of patients in a community nursing team is a complex role. Nevertheless, students may see this as a less onerous placement compared to leading a team with the delegation required on a hospital ward. This is clearly not the case as in the community the senior student is expected to undertake duties with much less direct supervision. In order for the mentor to assess the student's ability to function as an NQN in a community setting, she will need to supervise her activities from a distance with support being via telephone rather than in person. Consequently, her actions and decisions are undertaken with a much higher level of real autonomy.

References

Her Majesty's Stationery Office (HMSO) (2012) *The Human Medicines Regulations 2012: Schedule 16 Patient Group Directions*. London: HMSO. Statutory instrument available at: http://www.legislation.gov.uk/uksi/2012/1916/pdfs/uksi_20121916_en.pdf (accessed: 26 March 2017).

National Institute for Health and Care Excellence (NICE) (2014) *Pressure Ulcers: Prevention and Management*. London: NICE.

14 | **Effective delegation**

Overview

One of the commonest concerns of the newly qualified nurse (NQN) is over how to delegate care to others. Consequently, this is a skill that it would be best for you to learn as a senior student. This chapter examines this aspect of leadership and provides you with advice and guidance on delegating effectively and appropriately.

Introduction

Delegation is not an option, it is a responsibility. Without effective delegation a number of issues may arise that could result in patient harm. Delegation may be a complex phenomenon. A variety of nursing staff at differing grades can be challenging, and then when you factor in the interprofessional team as well, the challenges can multiply with differing aims, philosophies and responsibilities. Ultimately, however, through all this is the need to ensure there is effective patient safety, staff development, staff morale and motivation, and also communication.

As a qualified nurse, the Code (Nursing and Midwifery Council (NMC), 2015) clearly states that you are accountable for your acts and omissions, therefore you may wonder where you stand when delegating tasks. This is a conundrum especially when delegating to non-professionals who are not accountable to a professional body. This may be one of the reasons why staff are perhaps anxious about delegating but also why they may fail to delegate to others. The issue is that this option can be equally damaging to the individual being cared for as it will undoubtedly involve a member of staff trying to do too much and mistakes may happen, or they may become isolated as other staff cease to ask if they can help, identifying that the nurse does not trust anyone to carry our any other tasks. What needs to be acknowledged and clarified is that you can delegate tasks and you are accountable but they are still responsible. It is vital that you know the capabilities and competencies of those you are delegating to. In other words, ensuring the task has been performed to the required standard, and evaluating and checking it on completion is part of your responsibility as a delegator. Should the task be inadequate, then identifying why and producing an action plan as a result is advisable, as it may be down to a number of different reasons including poor practice that has been inherited, or simply misunderstanding. Another reason may be complacency and if this is the case then it is important to identify why the task should be carried out in the way you suggest.

How can delegation affect the healthcare environment?

'Selecting the right person to delegate to requires a corresponding leadership style. It is often assumed that delegation is a management role; however, recognising the talents and strengths of individuals . . . requires leadership qualities' (Bach and Ellis, 2011: 44). As identified, working in isolation when working in a team is inappropriate and can have negative effects on those who fail to delegate. Failing to delegate suggests mistrust and can negatively affect the morale of staff. This low morale can rapidly transfer to the majority of staff creating disharmony, a dysfunctional team approach and failures in care.

Delegation differs slightly from other supervision methods of staff you may be leading or managing. Similar to delegation is coaching, mentoring and directing. Each of these differ for the delegator or team leader. Directing tends to be associated with those who are relatively inexperienced; for example, a first-year student nurse with little experience in the health sector. Coaching may be for those who require motivation and have some limited knowledge, and involves short-term interventions in an attempt to motivate and engage. Mentoring allows the delegator to acknowledge a person's skill but supports them and encourages them to use their skill and redirect their commitment to the health provision. Delegating may be the most common in the healthcare setting where you hope that staff are committed to the care of the patients in your area and are competent to carry out the tasks or care required under your direction (Bach and Ellis, 2011).

Case study 14.1: Geoff

Geoff has been qualified for six years. He works on a medical ward that specializes in stroke. He believes that he should not be doing basic care and wants to attain a specialist nurse post as that is where he feels his skills lie. It is Sunday evening and he needs to do the drugs round. He delegates the enteral feeding in his bay to a first-year student nurse.

Reflection

- What should Geoff have done first?
- Why is this incorrect?
- What impact could it have on the student?
- What impact could this have on the patient?
- What impact could this have on the Trust?
- How could you best describe Geoff's attitude?

Ensuring the delegatee is safe and competent is vital in ensuring the safety of those in your care. The student was also vulnerable and may feel too afraid to speak up about their lack of knowledge. For a student nurse, assessment of competency is fundamental to their place on the educational programme and although the student would be at fault for not speaking up and discussing their lack of knowledge and competency, the staff nurse also has his accountability and responsibility to think about. As a qualified nurse we need to ensure that our skills and knowledge are used for the benefit of others. Geoff is clearly an experienced practitioner and rather than feeling that care is beneath him, he could make a real difference to more junior staff by teaching, mentoring, supporting and coaching staff around him. Being a specialist nurse does not devolve you of basic care and it certainly involves supporting and educating more inexperienced staff.

Other issues surrounding delegation are delegating to those who do not want to be delegated to. This is a relatively common anxiety for nurses, particularly student nurses in their final year of their programme where delegation must be undertaken in order to achieve the competency requirement and for new staff nurses who must delegate as part of their responsibilities as a staff nurse.

Reflection

- Think about when you have been delegating. What approaches did you take?
- What worked?
- When did it feel inappropriate or fail to achieve the outcome you wanted?

Keys to effective delegating lie in the philosophy of 'don't delegate something that you would not do yourself'. Negotiating and communicating the plan for the care required on the shift or the imminent issues can also help keep staff involved and rationalize why you are asking them to perform the task identified. Once you have finished what you are doing, going to the team and asking if they need you to help them finish the task can all help to create the team approach needed for a positive and healthy working environment. Everyone needs to feel valued and appreciated; delegating tasks and then going off to have your break or sitting chatting to other members of staff can be demoralizing to the staff being delegated to as they perceive a lack of respect and lack of consideration and care to them.

To lead!

Delegating and leading may go hand in hand. Effective leaders should be able to delegate efficiently. What one must consider however is that leadership does not just involve allocating jobs to others. It entails the sharing of a vision or goal, inspiring and motivating, and seeing the long-term view. There are a number of leadership styles that you can read about, but what is clear is that a *laissez-faire* style of leadership would be inappropriate in the healthcare environment. By this we mean a very relaxed and hands-off approach to leadership that could almost be misunderstood as a 'couldn't care' attitude. It has to rely on experienced, motivated staff to take action, but even these staff may require feedback and need to feel they are being led at times.

Case study 14.2: Liz

Liz is a very experienced ward sister. She had managed the nurse-led rehabilitation unit for 20 years and had very loyal staff. Many were experienced in the speciality and Liz was of the opinion that they knew what needed doing so she let them get on with it. She did value her staff but, as she knew they were competent and would probably tell her when there were problems, she did not ask them about the working environment, ask about their day or discuss ward developments or ideas for improving care. Staff began to become demoralized, felt they lacked direction and just did what they needed to do in their work. The routine became just that: a routine.

Reflection

- What style of leadership was Liz displaying?
- What impact is this having?
- How do you think this affects patient care and experience?
- What do you think will happen if this situation is not resolved?
- What could Liz and/or the staff do to remedy the situation?

Transformational leadership and delegation involves motivating and inspiring staff but in a way that develops them. This involves the leader as perhaps a mentor and coach and as someone who often achieves positive results in the workplace. This may be because staff feel valued as someone is investing in their development. Although Liz had faith in her staff, they need to be developed, to be motivated and to have some communication from Liz that helped them to know that they are valued. They also need to have insight and to be dynamic in order to avoid the static situation they have found themselves in.

Despite a cacophony of leadership styles and models to pick from, Martin (2000) suggests the following for success:

- Show that you value and respect your staff and this means having confidence in their ability.
- Provide opportunities for professional development.
- Be very clear about where their autonomy boundaries are to avoid frustration and lack of clarity.
- Keep staff informed and involved and this may involve discussing plans for the future and challenges ahead.
- Be patient in new developments and allow staff time and space to deliver the change. Perhaps giving approximate targets for completion can help guide and assist with your expectations. To go and take over when things are not progressing as you anticipate may destroy the investment you have made.

The Healthcare Leadership Model (National Health Service Leadership Academy, 2015) provides guidance and encourages reflection in preparing NHS staff for leadership. There are nine dimensions that should help to improve the quality and safety of health and care services. As a student nurse in your pre-transition phase this may seem irrelevant to you, but in actual fact it is very relevant. Understanding the theoretical underpinnings surrounding effective leadership can help you identify those very positive leadership behaviours that you may have, or will be witnessing in practice and this latter idea of role modelling can be extremely helpful to you.

Overall, identifying really positive behaviours and witnessing not so good behaviour will help you to develop your own leadership style that can have a very positive impact on the way you, and the team you are leading, work and deliver care.

It is extremely rewarding to lead a team that believes in you and who want to work together with such enthusiasm and motivation. There may still be times when morale can be low among some staff for a variety of reasons but if you continue to be effective in how you lead and seek to encourage, develop and motivate others, this should help to recover the equilibrium and staff may respond to the support available. If this kind of environment is developed, staff become more aware of their roles in the team, they become more knowledgeable and develop through their involvement.

Conclusion

Delegation is a skill that develops with confidence and experience. This does not mean that it is only done well when you have a certain level of knowledge and experience; it means it becomes more natural and less overwhelming as they increase. Effective delegation involves considering and respecting the team, and it involves effective and compassionate leadership. Through this style and philosophy of leadership, staff well-being may improve and so patient care is improved, thereby ensuring that the whole environment becomes a healthy one.

References

Bach, S. and Ellis, P. (2011) *Leadership, Management and Team Working in Nursing*. Exeter: Learning Matters.

Martin, V. (2000) Effective team leadership, *Nursing Management*, 10(5): 26–29.

National Health Service Leadership Academy (2011) *Clinical Leadership Competency Framework*. London: NHS.

National Health Service Leadership Academy (2015) *Healthcare Leadership Model*. Available at: http://www.leadershipacademy.nhs.uk/

15 Key skills of the staff nurse

> **Overview**
>
> The new registered nurse (RN) needs a set of skills in order to do their job effectively. Some of these have been described in previous chapters. This chapter provides you with the opportunity to reflect upon what the essential skills of a staff nurse are and how to incorporate them into the final placements of the programme in order to perfect them.

Introduction

In the nursing profession, the list of skills needed in order to be able to work as a registrant has been a controversial area of debate for some time. Chapter 10 explored the central concept of holistic care. This is a core tenet of the profession and this chapter is not intended as a challenge to that. Nevertheless, in order to understand and make sense of any profession, it is necessary to identify the constituent parts. Consequently, this chapter lists and examines the key skills of the staff nurse in order for the final year student to be able to practise and demonstrate the ability to practise as an RN.

Skills needed to be a staff nurse

Many of the skills needed in order to perform as a staff nurse have been examined in previous chapters, therefore much of this chapter can be seen as revision. However, it is important to try to identify what it is that is needed in practical terms to be able to be seen as a nurse worthy of registration. This can never be an exhaustive and all-inclusive list as there are variations as time progresses and in the context of different specialities and clinical settings. However, unless an attempt is made to quantify the role of the RN it can appear to be an unimaginable and therefore unachievable goal. The Nursing and Midwifery Council (NMC) have attempted to do this by producing a list of five essential skills clusters that encompass 42 skills (NMC, 2010):

- care, compassion and communication
- organizational aspects of care
- infection prevention and control
- nutrition and fluid management
- medicines management.

These clusters do appear sensible and have been in use since 2007. However, there are other ways of looking at practical nursing skills. Consequently, a list of practical skills that will be needed in your first job and seen as showing that you can perform as a newly qualified nurse (NQN) is provided in Box 15.1 in no particular order.

Box 15.1: Skills you will be required to use as a staff nurse

- Leadership, management, organization and delegation
- Infection control procedures
- Washing and dressing patients
- Teaching patients, students and staff
- Toileting patients and continence care
- Observation and interpretation of vital signs

  ○ Blood pressure; pulse; respiration; pulse oximetry; consciousness scales; blood glucose; urinalysis; central venous pressure; early warning scores; anthropometric measurements; body mass index

- Manual handling and mobilizing patients
- Communication, care and compassion

  ○ Psycho-social needs of patients through talking to them as a fellow human being; discussing and planning care with other nurses and the multidisciplinary team (MDT)
  ○ Providing clinical and social information for patients and those identified by the patient as trusted friends and family
  ○ Being an advocate for the patient
  ○ Literacy skills for written communication and documentation

- Understanding the roles of the MDT
- Medicines management including drug administration
- Feeding patients and supporting artificial nutrition
- Professional reflection – both on action and in action
- Critical analysis of research findings in order to assess best evidence-based practice (EBP)
- Wound dressing and aseptic technique
- Technology skills (see the next paragraph)

  ○ This could include the use of: cardiac monitor interpretation; ECG lead placement; urinary catheterization; intravenous infusion set up and monitoring; IV cannula insertion; bladder scanner diagnostics; wound drain and chest drain support; suction equipment; nasogastric tube insertion and maintenance; supporting physicians and other MDT members using technological treatments and therapies.
  ○ Pressure area care and monitoring

In the area of technology skills, this includes information technology (IT) and clinical technology. IT skills are now essential for a wide range of professions and nursing is no exception. Not only is the use of a computer necessary for documentation and communication but also hand-held devices are becoming the norm for drug administration and prescription and the recording of vital sign information. The specific set of clinical technological competencies necessary for an RN is highly debatable and is likely to vary depending on the speciality where the NQN starts their career. A complete list of technologies used would probably be far too long to provide. However, it could include those mentioned in Box 15.1.

The list above covers general skills and much more specific lists have been attempted. Some of the skills can and will be used by other staff but all of them fall within the role of the registered nurse (RN) depending on the circumstances of the job. The list of skills changes with time and context. Other staff registered at a lower level to RNs or unregistered but assessed as competent in some of these skills may take on any or all of those on the list. RNs may take on more advanced roles that will include other skills which have been associated with other professions in the past. For example, prescribing is becoming increasingly common for nurses and is one that may well be subsumed into the standard list in the near future.

Many of these skills will have been covered in the earlier stages of your course and you will have spent long hours in practice perfecting them. Consequently, they have not been covered in this book as it is about the final stages of your programme. As Crick *et al.* (2014) argue, this does not mean that these skills are unimportant or that they are beneath the role of the staff nurse to perform as some commentators have asserted. Nevertheless, as Manning argues:

> Many of the distressing stories we hear of inadequate care stem from patients not having help with basic needs such as assisting to the toilet, feeding and drinking. If you have 20 patients all being served lunch at the same time and 15 of them need help with eating, it's an impossible task.
>
> Manning (2013: 40)

As a result, it is often important for the RN to delegate those activities that other staff can do and reserve their activities to the jobs that only the RN can do or which it is more critical that an RN does. This is not being 'too posh to wash'; it is merely ensuring that everyone who needs to be washed is washed, fed and toileted or cared for in other important ways, and that the responsibilities that only the RN can do are also completed in a timely manner. These may include: administering medication, negotiating safe discharge, documenting the care provided to ensure continuity and explaining the complexities of the therapeutic regime to help the patient back to health. Overall it is the RN's responsibility to ensure that the holistic care of each of their patients is provided. This may, or may not, require the RN to physically do all of these activities but it does mean that they need to understand how they are done and to be able to delegate and monitor them effectively if they do not do them directly.

Case study 15.1: Dawn

You are Dawn, a senior student nurse and your mentor is assessing your ability to lead a team. Consequently, you have been practising taking charge of two bays of four patients each, making eight in total, for the last week on a hospital medical ward specializing in the care of patients with renal problems. The majority of the patients require nursing care for all of their activities of living (sometimes called 'full care') and are on a combination of medications to treat their long-term conditions. Every day since you started on the ward, you have taken responsibility for washing, dressing and helping with breakfast for two or three patients in addition to leading the team. You are very well practised in doing this and feel most comfortable when providing this fundamental care for your patients.

Your team consists of your mentor, who is an RN (Eve), a healthcare assistant (HCA) with 20 years' experience on the ward (Todd), and an assistant practitioner (AP) (May) who is qualified to take observations and to maintain wound dressings by the policies of the employing hospital. You know that the RN can provide any care required from the list above. The HCA can complete fundamental nursing care such as washing, feeding and toileting and the AP can undertake these duties and the two activities identified above. This morning the RN also has to administer medication to the patients on two other bays as well because the ward sister (Flo), who is responsible for those patients, has been required to do an audit with the matron. This means that your mentor will be unable to participate in any other activities due to the polypharmacy required to maintain patients with these complex conditions. You realize that you will not be able to be involved in washing and dressing the patients as your mentor will expect you to accompany her when administering drugs to your patients and then after that you will need to be available to attend an MDT meeting, which is scheduled for 8.30am regarding patients in your team. Consequently, you delegate the observations and wound dressings to the AP, May, and the fundamental care of five patients to the HCA, Todd, and the other three to May. You say that if they need assistance they should call on each other or on you if you are available. When he hears this, Todd says: 'Here we go. The student has got staff nurse-itis already; she's not even qualified yet and she's "too posh to wash". Not like Sister Flo; she's always prepared to roll up her sleeves and muck in.'

Reflection

1. Do you agree with Todd that nurses should always do fundamental care? Does it matter that Todd disagrees with Dawn's allocation of workload? What action should Dawn take in response to his opinions?
2. If Dawn did take primary responsibility for preparing one or two patients for the day would this be the best for the holistic care of all eight patients? Return to the list of skills provided above. As indicated, the RN can do and is responsible for all of these activities. Using your knowledge and experience, make a list of

a) which of these activities May can do and b) which Todd is permitted to perform?
3. Dawn is making decisions based on the best consequences for her patients. As a supernumerary student you can be involved in any part of the work activities, because the primary responsibility for the student is to enable their education leading to the ability to be a proficient RN. From a student perspective has Dawn made the right decision?

Reflection on skills already introduced

As can be seen in Case study 15.1, the skills learned at the beginning of the course are, arguably, as important to the RN as the more advanced skills that are taught towards the end of the programme. This is true even if as an RN you are forced, through lack of time, to delegate many of them to other staff. Where this happens you will need to be able to monitor the quality of care provided and to be able to offer advice and assistance when the person that you have delegated to needs assistance.

Case study 15.1 (*continued*): Dawn

During the shift above the AP, May, informs you that she has been unable to obtain a blood pressure reading for Mr Chang from the automated blood pressure monitor and is requesting you to take a manual blood pressure. She also thinks that he looks 'a bit grey'. You are in the middle of a discussion with the physiotherapist about another patient's discharge but you make your excuses and go to see Mr Chang. Mr Chang is alert and talking normally but his pulse is 120 beats per minute and you cannot obtain a blood pressure either. You ask May to call the doctor and the RN urgently, telling her to inform them that the early warning score is five, and you stay with Mr Chang (Royal College of Physicians (RCP), 2012).

Reflection

1. Was Dawn correct to leave the physio? Is this an emergency as Dawn seems to think?
2. Is Dawn's ability to take a manual blood pressure in question? Why do you think that she could not obtain a blood pressure measurement?
3. There are lots of things to do and seven other patients depending on Dawn. Why has she decided to stay with Mr Chang?

How to perfect your skills in the final placement

For the whole of your final placement you should be aiming to perfect and demonstrate your ability to function as an NQN. This requires courage as it would be very easy to carry on performing the fundamental skills perfected in the first stages of your course and fulfilling the fundamental care aspects of the RN skill set. The aspects of the nurse's role, therefore, which cannot be done by anyone else need to be focused upon. This will usually require you to assert your supernumerary status as some activities, such as patient group direction (PGD) supply and administration, are restricted by statute law to registrants and students are not permitted to administer them even under direct supervision. Drug administration of patient specific directions is often limited by employers to registrants and students are permitted to administer them only under their direct supervision. Similar restrictions will apply to other activities seen as more advanced and therefore it will be likely that you will only be able to observe or practise under direct supervision. Consequently, the best way to perfect these advanced skills is to make a list of the ones that you believe to be central to your needs when you start to work as an RN. This list can then form the basis of a discussion with your mentor to set learning objectives and a plan to achieve them during your placement. Remember that this will be your last chance to gain expertise in these skills prior to becoming a staff nurse when you will find it more difficult to obtain the necessary time and supervision that should be afforded to a supernumerary student.

Conclusion

The role of the nurse is often seen as nebulous and of unobtainable complexity to the senior student. Consequently, students may choose to continue limiting themselves to the role that they have perfected in their earlier stages of the course. Nevertheless, it is crucial to begin to gain a practical understanding and mastery of the specific skills required of the staff nurse during your final placement. With good communication skills, courage, confidence and persistence, it should be possible to practise these skills in your final placement when you are in the protected status of supernumerary student.

References

Crick, P., Perkinton, L. and Davies, F. (2014) Why do student nurses want to be nurses?, *Nursing Times*, 110(5): 12–15.

Manning, J. (2013) Making humanity matter, in Beer, G. (ed.) *Too Posh to Wash? Reflections on the Future of Nursing.* London: 2020 Health.

Nursing and Midwifery Council (NMC) (2010) *Standards for Pre-registration Nursing Education.* London: NMC.

Royal College of Physicians (RCP) (2012) *National Early Warning Score* (NEWS): *Standardising the Assessment of Acute-Illness Severity in the NHS.* Report of a Working Party. London: RCP.

16 Passing your sign-off mentor assessment

> **Overview**
>
> The Nursing and Midwifery Council (NMC) insists that your final placement experience is treated differently to all those that have gone previously. Your mentor has to be annotated on the local register as a sign-off mentor and this means that you have to face an even greater level of scrutiny and assessment than on other placements. This chapter provides a discussion of what is involved and offers advice and guidance on how to achieve the standards required by the sign-off mentor.

Introduction

Your final placement requires you to behave and practise with a level of competency deemed necessary for entry to the register. This means you are expected to work independently, to be able to carry out your role as a staff nurse by delegating tasks, leading a team, working with little direction, all the time behaving as someone who is about to transfer to the register. This does not mean, however, that you will be assessed as a staff nurse, but means that you need to be deemed a safe practitioner with adequate knowledge and understanding to allow you to be not only responsible for your actions, but also accountable for your actions. Although many of these skills will develop further once you have completed your transition, you still have to demonstrate a level of understanding and competency.

Once you embark on your management placement, you will have completed a full programme of theory and have undertaken a number of placements in a variety of areas. All this experience has led to this moment. This is the time when you consolidate it all and develop your confidence. There will still be doubts about your knowledge and understanding and, even as an experienced staff nurse, you may still hold doubts; this is reasonable. If you think you know everything, you are in danger of being overconfident and this, in itself, can carry risk. It is about recognizing, not only your skills and competency, but also your limitations. Once qualified it is acknowledged in the Code (NMC, 2015) that you should only work within the limits of your competency and knowledge, therefore the expectation is inherent in that requirement; that is, you will not know everything.

Sign-off mentor

While in this final placement, you will be assessed by a sign-off mentor. This mentor carries greater responsibility. It is not that the assessment itself is any more or less important than your previous assessments of competency, but this involves checking previous placement evaluations, potentially contacting previous mentors for verification or clarification, examining hours undertaken in practice, assessing placement experience and the range of that experience. It is a time-consuming process, but one that is vital as this may be the last assessment you undergo before embarking on your role as a staff nurse; therefore, one needs to be assured that you are assessed as safe and competent to practise independently. Sign-off mentors receive extra training input in order to prepare them for the role, identifying responsibilities in the process.

How do I cope?

It is difficult for any student in a placement area as you may feel under constant, close, scrutiny. The added pressure at this point is that it is the last placement and so much is being asked of you. Perhaps doing things that you may not have done before, having to use your judgement and work more independently, delegating, planning and leading may all be challenging you and taking you out of your comfort zone. Among the competencies required, things like your ability to delegate and lead are assessed in a summative manner and you may not have had as much experience or feel as confident as you would like regarding this. Allan *et al.* (2015) identified that as a newly qualified nurse (NQN), one of the major difficulties was delegation, therefore feeling anxious as a student nurse should, perhaps, be expected. What you need to consider and, indeed, remember is that you have worked extremely hard to get to this point and although you may not feel ready, you will in fact be ready because all the preparation will gradually, or maybe suddenly, make sense. Your mentor needs to know you are ready and the best way to let them know is to communicate effectively and openly about your plans, your concerns and your thought process.

Communication

When you are making decisions and using your judgement, relay your reasoning to your mentor as this will demonstrate your understanding and show that you have considered a number of options and issues before that final decision. It may impress your mentor, therefore it is well worth doing. This also applies to your reasoning surrounding delegating tasks, planning the day and prioritizing. To communicate this to your mentor is a really effective and safe way to get feedback from them and may give you some reassurance surrounding the decisions you have made. Having a discussion about your decisions can also be part of a learning opportunity as this may involve questions and answers so getting you to consider alternative routes or practice.

Case study 16.1: Gareth

Gareth was in his management placement. It was his fourth week and he had two bays of patients to manage. His mentor was part of his team alongside a healthcare assistant (HA) and a first-year student nurse. He took report and then considered the issues and priorities. He made a plan and then asked his mentor if they could listen to his rationale. He discussed his plan briefly outlining the student nurse's need for supervision and close guidance as well as her need to learn. He discussed the HA and the fact that she was experienced. He also indicated that they had two admissions and a discharge to deal with. He planned the activities and also considered the holistic needs of the patients including a patient whose relatives were in constant attendance due to their loved one's deteriorating condition. The mentor and Gareth discussed the situation in full and the mentor asked a question that Gareth responded to appropriately. The mentor praised Gareth's approach, particularly his considerations for the student nurse's well-being, the patient at the end of life and the HA.

Reflection

- How would you describe Gareth's leadership style?
- What benefits did his approach to communication with his mentor have?
- Are the time constraints regarding ward activity a problem for this approach?

Considering only the care activity and how it can be distributed should not be the only consideration. Gareth was thinking about staff well-being, patient safety and staff development and training. This consideration can help build more effective teamwork as it can foster enthusiasm, and also skills development (see Chapter 14 for further discussion).

In addition to demonstrating the ability to lead and delegate, you have to demonstrate proficiency in the other NMC competencies. Prior to the placement, it is worth considering how you could achieve them in the management placement, initially as an individual, then perhaps to discuss your plans with your sign-off mentor in your initial interview/discussion. In addition to your plans for meeting the competency in the domains, detailed discussions surrounding your own needs and expectations of the placement are paramount from the start (see Elsa's experience in Chapter 11). Other proactive means of preparing yourself for your placement include researching the placement speciality, the types of conditions and illnesses your patients may be suffering from. This can all aid your autonomous, compassionate, skilful and safe practice.

If you have a greater understanding surrounding the range of illnesses and conditions people may present with in your management area, then you may feel more prepared to deal with urgent issues in a safe and effective manner; and it may aid your decision making regarding prioritizing your care delivery. It will also help you practise holistically by understanding the conditions more fully and thinking about how this may affect the individual considering how the interprofessional team could contribute to the assessment, diagnostic reasoning, care planning, care delivery and evaluation.

What one must not forget is that professionalism is also paramount. In your haste to demonstrate skill, competency, delegation and leadership, you may be tempted to allow issues around professionalism to become a lower priority when these are just as essential, including the need to understand, acknowledge and respect our colleagues, to behave in a way that is appropriate for one who is about to enter the register as a qualified nurse, and to maintain your integrity. Being mindful surrounding others' needs is extremely important to enable effective team-working and safe patient care. Being good at delegating and understanding the impact a myocardial infarction has on a patient is not enough. Communicating effectively not only with patients but also with our colleagues is imperative.

Throughout all the assessment process, being compassionate with your patients and those around you is fundamental. Compassionate leadership, compassionate care and compassionate treatment of your colleagues should be considered essential when it comes to demonstrating you are fit to enter the nursing register.

Conclusion

Entering your management placement can feel daunting. You are not there as a staff nurse, you are being assessed as having a safe level of competency. Using effective communication with your sign-off mentor and to those around you, including allied health professionals, patients and nursing colleagues, can all aid in your successful completion. Preparing for your placement can alleviate some of the anxiety surrounding the unknown. It can help you to feel prepared around a number of areas, such as developing your understanding of patient conditions, routine medication management, ward philosophy and routine. Evidence-based practice (EBP) is essential and having the opportunity to examine the evidence surrounding care in the speciality you are embarking on is crucial in demonstrating your commitment and competency.

References

Allan, H. T., Magnusson, C., Horton, K., Evans, K., Ball, E., Curtis, K. and Johnson, M. (2015) People, liminal spaces and experience: understanding recontextualisation of knowledge for newly qualified nurses, *Nurse Education Today*, 35(2): e78–83.

Bondy, N. K. (1983) Criterion-referenced definitions for rating scales in clinical education, *Journal of Nursing Education*, 22(9): 376–382.

Nursing and Midwifery Council (NMC) (2015) *The Code*. London: NMC.

17 Applying for and obtaining your first registered nurse position

Overview

Once the programme is passed in theory and practice, the next most important stage is obtaining the right position. This chapter examines the evidence to discover where jobs are likely to be available for newly qualified nurses (NQNs). It considers the application strategies available to you and what to look out for in a good, supportive employer.

Introduction

Although it is important you find the right job for you, it may be that, as you complete your programme, either the area you want to move to does not take recently qualified staff, or there may be no vacancies. It is reasonable to take a different post for a period of time, perhaps until you have completed your preceptorship and then to think about where you want to be in the future or start trying to attain your dream job.

There are anxieties in applying for your first job and these range from completing the application through to the interview process and starting the job. Anxieties can revolve around which job to choose if you have more than one offer and all the other anxieties about transition to registration; for example, time management, delegation and supervision (Allan *et al.*, 2016; Magnusson *et al.*, 2017). You need to attain employment in order for you to develop as a registered nurse (RN) and no matter where you work, you are likely to gain experience and consolidate your learning. It is often a case of weighing up the merits of the offers. There may be anxieties about all the posts offered but it is about trying to ascertain which one is the most likely to lead you to where you want to be?

Case study 17.1: Harriet

Harriet is due to qualify in September. She eventually would like to work in an oncology unit. She has applied for three posts. One post is in the community hospital close to where she lives and therefore would be ideal for her travel time. The other two posts are in the acute trust: one on a medical ward specializing in respiratory conditions and the second on a surgical ward specializing in colorectal surgery. She is really anxious regarding which post she should take. Her last placement was on the medical ward and she really enjoyed the pace, she enjoyed the speciality and the ward had a very dynamic team. The surgical ward had a good team with a specialist nurse on site and the majority of patients having surgical intervention had a cancer diagnosis. She went to see her personal tutor to discuss her concerns. The personal tutor would not tell her which post to accept but suggested she plot her career pathway, examine the advantages and disadvantages of each option and discuss the options for professional development with the each of the ward managers. She also suggested she should contact the careers team at the university for further help and support.

Reflection

- Which post do you think she should take, and why?
- Can you see the merit of speaking to the ward manager?
- What about the university careers service?

It is difficult being faced with a number of job opportunities, but also being faced with only one option that does not appeal can be equally difficult. In nursing, it is often about seeing where you want to be in the future and thinking about how you get there from where you are right now rather than just thinking about now. This may be a more positive approach. It is a career rather than just a job, and in looking forward and progressing, although not for everyone, nursing seems to hold numerous opportunities. Nurses do not necessarily have to be constrained and remain in the same environment no matter what the employment situation, even if it means casting your eyes further geographically. The other issue you need to consider is where you find the right job.

Searching for a job

Finding the right job for you is a challenge, and, as suggested earlier, it may not happen the first time. Your university may have departments that are there to help you with things like CV writing and applications, and may have contacts and information regarding job fairs where you have the chance to see what the current employment offers and opportunities are. At job fairs there is also the chance to chat with employers and find out more about the organization that may give an indication of the working philosophy and how you may be supported. You need to feel that you are going somewhere that will be supportive and responsive to your needs. Phillips *et al.* (2014) examined experiences and needs of graduate nurses during the transition to RN and, as anticipated, greater support was associated with improved transition experience. Consequently, it would be advisable to try to determine that the environment is one where staff adopt a more encouraging and coaching approach to help and aid a more seamless and less stressful transition.

Other options are through your university lecturers. Often, if they have good links with clinical practice, potential employers who want to recruit newly qualified staff will often contact lecturing staff to advertise their interest. This does not mean that the staff advocate you work in any particular environment or with any specific employer; they give you the information to help you attain the post you desire.

Some Trusts have clearing activities that mean at times when they know NQNs are ready for employment, they save a number of jobs and offer mass interviews to attract candidates. They then offer the post to the best candidates. This often means going in for a general post; that is, not site-specific. You may find out at the interview what the area is but it may be that this is done after the interview. The problem is that you may get an area you do not want, but if this happens, all is not lost; there may be the opportunity to negotiate.

A further option is to check places where jobs are advertised. Places like the nursing press can give you up-to-date vacancies and also websites like National Health Service (NHS) Jobs will often give you a greater understanding surrounding posts around the region or in the UK. The difficulty is that often the application asks for your Nursing and Midwifery Council (NMC) pin number that you may not have at the point of application. If this is the case you could contact the human resources department of the employer and ask their advice. It may be that they are looking for experienced nurses but, depending on the employment climate, they may need to take NQNs; therefore, they may take your application without a pin number.

A further option is an agency post. This allows you to get a wider range of experience in a number of healthcare settings. If this is what you need with regard to your future ambitions, then this may be the right choice for you. Some NQNs are fearful of getting a permanent post and not liking the practice area, especially if they have not had any experience in that particular area. Working with an agency can give you a real feel of differing practice and environments but you must be mindful that working cohesively in a team may be challenging when you are only going for one shift, and also it is only a 'taster' – you are not going to build expertise in that area after just one or two shifts. It may be similar to going to a new placement as a student each time and, although you are not assessed, staff will be observing your practice and ensuring you are competent. It may be that you need something to bridge a gap; for example, waiting to move oversees, pending your application to join the armed forces. Joining an agency to gain that wide range of experience can be beneficial.

The application

It is paramount that you seek help in this application process if you are a novice. Even as an experienced applicant, getting another person's view can be beneficial. Careers advisers at your university or personal tutors can be really helpful and give you some good advice. They will have been in your position and can relay their often vast experience surrounding applications and job hunting.

You have to get your application right and this means ensuring that your application meets all the essential criteria on the job specification. This should help to guarantee you an interview. Employers are not looking for extensive dialogue in your supporting statement, they are looking for succinct information that suggests you are exactly what they need. Your personal statement needs to stand out. Make yourself unique compared to the other applicants. This can be achieved by relaying short clinical experiences so rather than saying, 'I am a good communicator', you can relay a situation where you supported the medical staff when a patient was having bad news delivered, and you stayed with them afterwards and answered their questions and gave them time to comprehend the news. This does not only provide evidence surrounding your communication skills, but also suggests you may be compassionate and patient. Recalling anecdotes like this can also be helpful in the interview itself as it makes you memorable.

Giving yourself enough time is paramount when completing your application. A rushed application may mean that you fail to give a considered personal statement, or it could contain errors, and this may result in you being rejected. Do not wait to submit it near the closing date; if you have internet connection issues or there are other problems, you may miss the deadline. Make sure you proofread your work thoroughly and ask someone else to. Finally, submit it and fingers crossed you have already started to impress them!

The waiting

This can be a difficult time, particularly if it is the job you really want. This is not a time for sitting and waiting however. You can make the most of this time to research the area more fully. Going in prepared demonstrates your commitment and enthusiasm but also it can suggest that you are professional and are taking this opportunity seriously. Research can be done about the employer; for example, a Trust or private organization. You can look at the community it serves and the types of treatment it gives, and this can give you the opportunity to read up about specific conditions as well. Another useful activity is going to visit the placement area. Some employers feel this is important and demonstrates interest and again that vital commitment. One would question why anyone would turn up for an interview to a place they had never been to or seen. If it is an international job then one may be forgiven but for a job in the same country it is questionable.

The interview

Your opportunity is there waiting for you. You need to wow the interviewers. You need to stand out, but for the right reasons! Start with thinking about situations that demonstrate your leadership and delegation skills, communication, compassion and teamworking abilities. These are all key qualities that a nurse needs and it will stop you just listing the qualities, which, if done as a list, become less believable. By preparing to talk about various situations, then, if you are nervous, which is a perfectly normal response to an interview, worrying about having nothing to say or your mind going blank becomes less of an issue. You can always tell one of the stories about a situation that you had to respond to and this will usually be relayed with some sort of emotion, and this becomes more meaningful to an interviewer but also, more importantly, you become more memorable; for example, 'the one that told us about the time they . . .'

Dress is important too. You do not want to feel uncomfortable in the interview. Men need to think about their shirt and ensuring it is not too tight so that it becomes gaping. Smart clothing suggests you really want to make a good impression and you have taken the time to prepare. It demonstrates some respect to your interviewers too. Women should try to wear clothing that is not too short as they may end up trying to pull the skirt or dress down in the interview as it will ride up as they seat themselves. Once again, a blouse or dress that is too tight will make you feel uncomfortable and potentially your interviewer too!

The way you answer questions and engage with the interviewers is vital. You can dress well, prepare well, have visited the area but if you do not display enthusiasm and commitment or answer questions as fully as you can then all your efforts may be in vain. Think about the idea of working there as they are interviewing you and you should feel a knot of excitement, this may come across then as you are answering their questions.

If they are asking multi-layer questions that require more than one answer then you can ask them to repeat the question. An interviewer expects this and they also expect you to be nervous, so do not worry about a nervous rash or the odd stammer. It is important that you give the answer they are looking for, so checking you have heard them correctly is paramount. If there is information in the question then it is likely that it is relevant to your answer, and this is particularly the case when there are clinical scenario-based questions.

If it is a situation you have not dealt with, or a patient with a condition you are not familiar with, the best option for you would be to say, 'I am sorry but I have not cared for someone with this particular condition or seen this performed'. You can then add that you would ask another member of staff for advice, or, if it is a task, then perhaps get them to do the task with you observing. What you are demonstrating here is that you recognize your limitations, but also, that you are keen to learn. They may be asking you about something that needs extra training to undertake; for example, a peripherally inserted catheter (PICC) line. To say something like 'well I have not dealt with one before but I would get a syringe and flush it with saline . . .' would be unsafe and demonstrate a lack of awareness surrounding recognizing your limitations.

Lastly, when they ask if you have any questions, you need to have at least one, but perhaps no more than three, as this may be time consuming and you should have had most of your questions answered on your visit to the area. As an NQN, asking about preceptorship is always useful and demonstrates your enthusiasm for learning. Questions like, 'how quick can I get a sister's post?' Or 'what is the salary?' are perhaps not the right questions to be asking at the interview. When this is over, take a deep breath, stand up and shake their hands, thanking them for the interview and remember to smile!

The waiting, again!

Once again, the wait. Ensure that if you gave them your mobile number it is charged and switched on with volume control up. You do not want to miss that vital call. When the phone rings, remain calm and listen. If you have been successful, you can tell them you are thrilled and thank them. If you have not, then you can ask them for some feedback. They may give you some information over the telephone or they may offer written or verbal feedback face to face. Either way it is important for you to understand why you have not been successful in order to prepare for your next interview. Do not be too downhearted, it perhaps was not meant to be, but also you are gaining vital interview experience, so try to see it as a positive rather than a negative. Sometimes it is not that you are not good enough, it is that they may feel you will not fit into the team. Managers should consider the team members and the personality types in order to ensure the team remains functional (Bach and Ellis, 2011).

Conclusion

Although anxiety-provoking, this is an all-important and invaluable experience. You need to attain a job and the more prepared you are and committed you are to getting a job, the more successful you are likely to be. Seeking help with applications, researching the area and thinking about what you have to offer them, including your personal qualities, can all help to get you your dream job.

References

Allan, H., Magnusson, C., Evans, K., Ball, E., Westwood, S., Curtis, K., Horton, K. and Johnson, M. (2016) Delegation and supervision of healthcare assistants' work in the daily management of uncertainty and the unexpected in clinical practice: invisible learning among newly qualified nurses, *Nursing Inquiry*, 23(4): 377–385.

Magnusson, C., Allan, H., Horton, K., Johnson, M., Evans, K. and Ball, E. (2017) An analysis of delegation styles among newly qualified nurses, *Nursing Standard*, 31(25): 46–53.

Phillips, C., Kenny, A., Esterman, A. and Smith, C. (2014) A secondary data analysis examining the needs of graduate nurses in their transition to a new role, *Nurse Education Practice*, 14(2): 106–111.

Registration (or why you should be confident and resilient as a registered nurse in your first post as a newly qualified nurse)

18 | How to become a valuable part of the team

Overview

One of the most important measures of a successful newly qualified nurse (NQN) is that the rest of the team value their input. This chapter provides insights into what things you can do as a new registered nurse (RN) to show your value at an early stage. It discusses the reasons why there might be difficulty in doing this in some teams and that this is just a product of you being a new starter.

Introduction

Fitting into a community is a basic human need, and whenever a new member of a team arrives it potentially can upset the dynamic of the existing team. Consequently, when you start as an NQN in your first position, you will want to become a part of the community as quickly as practicable. However, that does not mean putting up with whatever the prevailing culture is no matter what; therefore, when to speak out is dealt with in Chapter 19. In this chapter it is assumed that the existing workplace community is reasonably supportive.

What things a new RN can do in order to show their value at an early stage

The NQN entering the workplace should be welcomed as a new professional able to bring their skills, knowledge, compassion and empathy to it. They will not have the experience of other staff but will have the most up-to-date evidence-based education. This is logically the case, even if other members of the team have been qualified for short periods of time. Even in a practical sense this will make a difference as healthcare progresses so rapidly. Consequently, the value of the NQN is not only in being an additional pair of hands, even though this should not be underestimated in times of nursing shortage. The things that preceptors say they value in NQNs are a new perspective and a willingness and enthusiasm to care and to learn in their speciality. In our research into supporting the experiences of NQNs, preceptors indicated that NQNs were at the stage in their career where they had 'passed their driving test' and consequently, 'were just about to start to learn to drive' (Whitehead *et al.*, 2016). In other words, completion of pre-registration education gave NQNs the licence to start learning their profession. The idea of an ongoing continuum of learning as a professional is in line with Benner's (1984) 'from novice to expert' stages of clinical competency:

- novice
- advanced beginner
- competent
- proficient
- expert.

The stage that any RN is on in this continuum will depend on the speciality and workplace as well as the proximity to the point of registration. This willingness to learn in their first job as an RN is valued by others in the profession and the NQN should show that they are eager to learn the ropes through questioning, practising and through self-directed study of the common medical, psychological and social conditions of their patients.

Two theoretical ways of looking at the issues related to becoming a valuable member of the team are used here. These are the stages of small group development (Tuckman and Jensen, 1977) and the functional roles of group members (Benne and Sheats, 1948). These will be examined alongside the experiences of NQNs as relayed in our own and others' research projects and reflection on professional experience (Whitehead *et al.*, 2013; Whitehead *et al.*, 2016).

It is worth emphasizing that the newly arrived NQN should seek to become a valued team member as soon as possible. This is because, first, in order to deliver good nursing care to patients, a collaborative approach involving many individual practitioners with a multiplicity of roles working together is required. If the nursing and inter-professional team trust and value the nurse's involvement, then patient care will be improved. Second, it makes the life of the individual more pleasant and motivating if the community of practitioners around them value and respect their input. The NQNs in our systematic literature review and our research project indicated that there was an initial stage of uncertainty when they were unsure of their role and the local workplace community unsure of their ability. In order to show their value to the ward as soon as possible the NQN would do well to consider the theoretical constructs cited above. These are now expanded upon.

Tuckman and Jensen's (1977) stages of small group development can be summarized as:

- Forming
- Storming
- Norming
- Performing
- Adjourning.

The conceptual framework put forward is that each group formed to produce an outcome goes through these stages. The outcome in this case is the care of patients in the clinical workplace where NQNs find themselves. The theory is designed for groups forming together of new members at the same time. However, it can be adapted from the individual's viewpoint whenever a new member joins the team. Using this framework it would suggest that the experience of the NQN joining the team would progress as follows.

Forming

The NQN joins the team which therefore forms a new team. The initial forming stage is ideally an experience of welcoming and understanding from the existing team (Whitehead *et al.*, 2016). Unfortunately, it could also be one of incivility and professional sabotage (Maben *et al.*, 2006; Halpin, 2015). If it is the latter, and even with the former to a lesser extent, this is likely to lead to the next stage in the framework.

Storming

This is an emotional situation in which the NQN has to work out their new role and position within the team. The storming stage can be particularly difficult for the NQN because, unless they have knowledge of the research that suggests this is just a step in the process, they will perceive this as the way things will be as an RN.

Norming

After a while, the NQN and the nursing team will 'learn the ropes' and be able to understand the social structures of the workplace. They will also begin to get to grips with their own professional expectations. Maben *et al.* (2006) argue that this is not necessarily a good thing if the organization is not focused on individualized care and the local professional expectations are at odds with those of the NMC.

Performing

If the workplace is professional and well organized, it should be possible to move on to performing. This is the ideal destination of any team and for the individual within it. In this stage the team is performing its caring duties at the optimum level and the individual is able to provide the best nursing care because they have gained the skills to perform their role and have the trust of the team to do so.

Adjourning

This final stage is reached when the individual leaves the team or the team is disbanded because the purpose of it is no longer required.

This theoretical framework was based on Tuckman and Jensen's review of existing research literature. It is also supported by the experiences of NQNs in our systematic review (Whitehead *et al.*, 2013) and primary research (Whitehead *et al.*, 2016) and that of others (Maben *et al.*, 2006; Halpin, 2015). However, it is worth remembering that there is nothing inevitable about any theoretical structure no matter how well supported by the empirical evidence. Nevertheless, this framework can be useful to you as an NQN. If you keep it in mind when considering the feelings that you have or the behaviour of your colleagues, you will be able to console yourself in challenging periods that this is a journey through the stages above rather than a fixed state.

Why other members of the team may not value your work

Case study 18.1 examines the experience of an NQN.

Case study 18.1: Medications administration

You have started work on your first job as a staff nurse on a medical ward in an acute hospital. You have been welcomed into the team and provided with an induction programme and a named preceptor to support you during your first few months after qualifying. Part of the induction was an assessment of your ability to administer medications to patients that you found quite stressful but passed well. You now have your NMC personal identification number (PIN) and are allowed to administer drugs. However, it takes you twice as long as the other nurses to administer the medications to your patients and you have to keep looking things up in the British National Formulary (BNF). Most of the staff are supportive and tell you that 'it takes as long as it takes and the important thing is to be safe'. Unfortunately, one long-standing RN makes it clear to you that she thinks that you are too slow and that in her day nurses could administer drugs quickly before they were qualified.

Reflection

1. How do the theoretical frameworks help your understanding of this scenario?
2. Do you think that the critical RN is likely to be accurately remembering her NQN experience?
3. Do you think that you would be able to increase the speed in which you are able to administer medications safely? If so, why?

In the scenario above, it is clear that one of the nurses does not value the work of the NQN, seeing the NQN as being too slow. It is desirable to complete activities such as administering medications and other areas of patient care both efficiently and safely in order to be able to provide the optimum level of care to all patients. However, you will be slower as an NQN at conducting any procedure that requires the acquisition of complex skills and is highly safety critical for patients, such as drug administration. Speed at conducting these roles can only be safely achieved through having a good knowledge of the expected routes, dose, actions, side effects and contraindications. In addition, the nurse needs to know the nature of the conditions that necessitate the medications administered. As each NQN is aware, the consequences of error can be fatal (World Health Organization (WHO), 2008). Consequently, any criticism of NQNs for being too slow is usually ill advised and unfair.

If the employer is following the evidence-based advice indicated in Chapter 25, the critical nurse above should be in the minority as the culture of the workplace should be supportive. However, there is no guarantee of this. Your individual actions in dealing with this will rely in part on your ability to weather this stage in your career through the use of resilience as discussed in Chapter 24. However, if the incivility from other members of the team is too great to withstand, then consider either discussing this with the culprits or with your preceptor or line manager.

You should aim to become more efficient in all roles for the reasons given above. Safely increasing speed will come with practice as you become more dexterous and through studying the conditions and medications related to the specific medical speciality of the workplace. If you attempt to work at a faster pace without these building blocks, then it is likely that avoidable errors will be made.

Benne and Sheats (1948) suggested a set of 26 different roles that can be played by members of a group. These roles are divided into three categories:

- Task roles: getting the work done
- Personal and/or social roles: positive functioning of the team
- Dysfunctional and/or individualistic roles: disruptive to team purpose and unity.

These are not fixed for all time for each individual and are likely to vary dependent on the circumstances in which each person finds themselves. However, it may be helpful to see the members of the team fitting into these roles. The psychological and social underpinning of a team member for choosing their role (e.g. dysfunctional) is difficult if not impossible to determine and it is likely to have nothing to do with your own activities even if it appears to be directed at you. It is easy to prove this, as the reaction of different members of the team to the same behaviour on your part will be different, dependent on the role they are playing at the time.

Conclusion

You will become a valuable member of the team if you apply yourself to studying the common conditions, treatments and routines of the workplace. You should also apply yourself to practising the skills and activities in order to become proficient. If the other staff can observe you doing this, then they should in fairness value you as a team member.

References

Benne, K. D. and Sheats, P. (1948) Functional roles of group members, *Journal of Social Issues*, 4(2): 41–49.
Benner, P. E. (1984) *From Novice to Expert : Excellence and Power in Clinical Nursing Practice.* Menlo Park, CA: Addison-Wesley Publishing, Nursing Division.
Halpin, Y. (2015) *Newly Qualified Nurse Transition: Stress Experiences and Stress-Mediating Factors – a Longitudinal Study.* PhD thesis. London Southbank University.
Maben, J., Latter, S. and Macleod Clark, J. (2006) The theory-practice gap is alive and unwell: the impact of professional-bureaucratic work conflict on the experiences of newly qualified nurses in the UK, *Journal of Advanced Nursing*, 55(4): 465–477.
Tuckman, B. and Jensen, M. (1977) Stages of small group development revisited, *Group and Organization Studies*, 2(4): 419–427.
Whitehead, B., Owen, P., Holmes, D., Beddingham, E., Simmons, M., Henshaw, L., Barton, M. and Walker, C. (2013) Supporting newly qualified nurses in the UK: a systematic literature review, *Nurse Education Today*, 33(4): 370–377.
Whitehead, B., Owen, P., Henshaw, L., Beddingham, E. and Simmons, M. (2016) Supporting newly qualified nurse transition: a case study in a UK hospital, *Nurse Education Today*, 36: 58–63.
World Health Organization (WHO) (2008) *Learning from Error – Video and Booklet.* Available at: http://www.who.int/patientsafety/education/vincristine_download/en/

19 When to speak out

Overview

Being accepted by other members of a team is important, but you must also be prepared to speak out if you do not believe appropriate care is being provided. This chapter discusses the ethical and legal practicalities of when and where to raise concerns.

Introduction

This chapter considers when to speak out about inappropriate care or other professional issues. This is an obligation that you have as a nurse, which the Nursing and Midwifery Council (NMC) (2015a) describes as 'your role in raising concerns'. This professional duty can involve speaking out against colleagues or even your employers and is not an easy part of the responsibilities of the nurse. However, as the Chief Nursing Officer for England has indicated, nurses must have the courage to do the right thing and to speak up when things are wrong (Cummings and Bennett, 2012). In addition to being something that nurses must do, it is also something that when necessary, nurses want to feel supported in doing (Whitehead and Barker, 2010). It is hoped that this chapter helps you feel more confident to take action by providing you with a deeper understanding of what you need to do and when.

When to speak out if you do not believe appropriate care is being provided

At an everyday level it is a personal decision whether to go along with the existing ways of doing things or whether to try to change things in line with what you believe to be the best evidence-based approach. With most things, if the practice in your first workplace appears to be at odds with what you have been taught in your pre-registration course, it is best to do some research to check that your understanding of best practice is the most up to date and evidence based (see Chapter 3). If your alternate understanding appears to be right, then you should discuss this with your preceptor in the first instance. However, be realistic in your aspirations. If the benefit is slight and may be debatable, then be prepared for possible resistance if trying to change other RNs' practice.

If it is a more important issue there is clear guidance to nurses on when to speak out from the NMC (2015a) and the Department of Health (DH) (2014). There are two central ideas behind this, which are summarized as the following:

1. Any activities that are leading to detrimental care should be illuminated, stopped and learned from.
2. Nurses should use the structures set up by employers and local authorities to raise their concerns and only if these fail to be acted upon should the nurse consider whistleblowing outside of the organized structure.

The DH (2014) guidance and the NMC (2015a) list possible forms of abuse as follows:

- physical abuse
- domestic violence
- sexual abuse
- psychological abuse
- financial or material abuse
- modern slavery
- discriminatory abuse
- organizational abuse
- neglect and acts of omission
- self-neglect.

The nurse should not feel constrained by this list as it is designed to be a way of indicating that abuse can take many forms. It is also worth remembering that the concerns you may feel it is appropriate to raise could be related to abuse of staff or inappropriate or dishonest workplace practices.

Case study 19.1: Community staff nurse

You are working as a community staff nurse. During your visit to a patient she asks you to take her to the toilet as her usual carer, her son, has taken the opportunity to go out for a few minutes while you are visiting. When you get her into the toilet she says that she cannot 'go' and that her son usually punches her in the stomach to help her. You ask her to repeat what she has said and she confirms this.

Reflection

1. Based on the above list of possible forms of abuse, is this abuse?
2. Do you consider that it is safe to leave your patient in the care of her son?
3. What action should you take? Should it be reported and if so, to whom?

The guidance indicates that nurses should be proportionate in their response to any suspected abuse and should consider whether it is intentional or unintentional. These can be difficult judgements to make and in the case above it would be sensible for the registered nurse (RN) to discuss this disclosure with a more senior colleague in the first instance.

In Case study 19.1 it is a member of the patient's family who has been unwittingly identified as a potential, if probably misinformed and unintentional, abuser. However, it may be even more difficult if the apparent abuser is a member of staff who you work with or even your line manager. Case study 19.2 provides an example of this dilemma.

Case study 19.2: Nursing home

You are working in a nursing home. During your shift you walk around the residents' rooms and find that one person, with a diagnosis of advanced dementia, is sitting in her chair in her room with her wrists tied to the chair arms with bandages. You know that this resident has had her mental capacity assessed and been found to lack the capacity to make decisions for herself. You ask one of the carers about this and she tells you that the nursing home manager has instructed that anyone who has a tendency to wander should be restrained in this way 'for their own good'.

Reflection

1. Considering the list above, is this abuse?
2. Do you consider that it is safe to leave your patient in the care of this nursing home?
3. What action should you take? Should it be reported and if so, to whom?

Read the NMC guidance on raising concerns (2015a). Have you changed your view on whether she should have raised this and with whom after reading this?

In Case study 19.2 it would appear fairly straightforward that abuse is taking place. The patient lacks capacity in the terms of the *Mental Capacity Act* (Her Majesty's Stationery Office (HMSO), 2005). However, it is less obvious who to talk to about this in the first instance than in Case study 19.1. The straightforward answer to this is that if you are concerned for the immediate safety of individuals in your care, you should contact either the local council contact for adult safeguarding or the police.

All of the advice above relates to using the raising concerns framework (NMC, 2015a). This is the case even when you report outside of the employers' internal structure to adult safeguarding in the local council or the police. However, concerned individuals, including nurses, have sometimes found it appropriate to appeal directly to the media in order to blow the whistle on an institution for poor or deliberately abusive care. Perhaps the most well-known instance of an RN doing this was Margaret Haywood. This brave nurse became an undercover reporter for the BBC and investigated a hospital ward using a hidden camera. The poor care that she uncovered was shocking and highlighting this on national TV led to improvements in care at the hospital. However, she was initially reported to the NMC and struck off the register for breaching confidentiality. The NMC allowed her back onto the register after a nine-month public campaign for reinstatement. In her interview for the Whistleblower Interview Project (2012), Ms Haywood indicated that legal counsel she had taken prior to disclosing the evidence via the BBC *Panorama* programme had advised her not to do this. Nevertheless, she felt morally obliged to report this for the good of her patients. The next section explores the ethical and legal practicalities further.

The ethical and legal practicalities of when and where to raise concerns

Law regarding raising concerns

The main legislation covering the issue of raising concerns for nurses are the *Public Interest Disclosure Act*, 1998 (HMSO, 1998), *Mental Capacity Act*, 2005 (HMSO, 2005) and the *Care Act*, 2014 (HMSO, 2014). Advice on the legal practicalities can be obtained from your employer, your trade union or from independent organizations such as Public Concern at Work (2013). The NMC has a legal responsibility to protect the public and maintain a nursing register. Consequently, as an RN you are also subject to the statutory legislation that governs NMC registrants (Dimond, 2015). As stated in the previous section, if you have immediate concerns for the safety of your patient, then you should contact the police or the local council adult safeguarding office. If not, then the employer's procedures for raising concerns should be followed if there are any. All good employers should have this.

Ethics regarding raising concerns

It is the professional moral duty of nurses to raise concerns when appropriate. This is clear in the NMC Code and its guidance on raising concerns (NMC, 2015a; NMC, 2015b). The NMC provide some clear advice on the professional ethical rules related to this and that is helpful. However, this was not all that Ms Haywood was referring to when she said that she felt morally obliged to report on what she saw as abuse of patients. Ethics is the study of what is good or bad, right or wrong. It is a philosophical rather than a scientific discipline and therefore relies on logic rather than empirical evidence to produce rules to follow. Different philosophical approaches can lead to varying advice on deciding whether an action is the right or wrong one with a good or bad outcome.

The main ethical frameworks used in nursing and healthcare ethics are deontology or duty-based ethics; utilitarian or consequence-based ethics and the four ethical principles approach to biomedical ethics (Edwards, 2009; Beauchamp and Childress, 2012). These are vast and complex philosophical arenas that can be explored in more depth with further reading. These are briefly discussed in Chapter 12. However, it is worth considering these briefly here:

- Deontology describes ways of deciding whether an action is right or wrong by making a rule that you always follow.
- Utilitarianism bases decision making on what the outcome of the particular action is likely to be without any underpinning rule other than the greatest happiness of the greatest number.

Neither can claim to be the best way of approaching decision making and it is probably best to consider your actions from both approaches before deciding which course of action to take.

The four principles approach of Beauchamp and Childress (2012) has become dominant in bio-medical and nursing ethics. The four principles can be considered using both of the overall underpinning ethical frameworks indicated above. The four principles are:

- Autonomy: the patient has the freedom to choose what happens to themselves.
- Beneficence: the practitioner should seek to do good when treating the patient.
- Non-maleficence: the practitioner should try to do no harm to the patient.
- Justice: the patient should be treated without any unfair discrimination.

Beauchamp and Childress (2012) argue that these principles should all be seen as equally important. However, other ethicists have argued that the principle of autonomy should be given more weight than the others (Edwards, 2009). In practice these are useful principles to check whatever action you are taking as an RN whenever there are difficult decisions to be made. They can certainly be used when deciding whether to raise a concern and in what way.

Conclusion

The decision to speak out is sometimes a difficult one and sometimes very straightforward. With minor issues it is something to consider and to make sure that you are on solid ground before trying to change the rest of the team's hearts and minds. If it is an issue of abuse, then there is now clear advice and structures of support to refer to and you should ensure that you know what to do before any major issue arises. Nevertheless, even with the current level of support and legislative guidance, there are still difficult moral and professional decisions to be made. Make sure that whenever possible you can discuss the decision you make with the appropriate person, such as the local council or police or the senior colleague depending on the situation, as described above. Remember, it is a privileged position to be an RN and with that privilege comes the responsibility to raise concerns when appropriate.

References

Beauchamp, T. L. and Childress, J. F. (2012) *Principles of Biomedical Ethics*, 7th edn. New York and Oxford: Oxford University Press.

Cummings, J. and Bennett, V. (2012) *Developing the Culture of Compassionate Care: Creating a New Vision for Nurses, Midwives and Care-givers*. London National Health Service (NHS).

Dimond, B. (2015) *Legal Aspects of Nursing*, 7th edn. Harlow: Pearson Education.

Edwards, S. D. (2009) *Nursing Ethics: A Principle-based Approach*, 2nd edn. Basingstoke: Palgrave Macmillan.

Department of Health (DH) (2014) *Care and Support Statutory Guidance Issued under the Care Act 2014*. [Online]. Available at: https://www.gov.uk/government/uploads/system/uploads/attachment_data/file/315993/Care-Act-Guidance.pdf

Her Majesty's Stationery Office (HMSO) *Public Interest Disclosure Act* (1998) London: HMSO.

Her Majesty's Stationery Office (HMSO) *Mental Capacity Act* (2005). London: HMSO.

Her Majesty's Stationery Office (HMSO) *Care Act* (2014). London: HMSO.

Nursing and Midwifery Council (NMC) (2015a) *Raising Concerns: Guidance for Nurses and Midwives*. London: NMC. Available at: https://www.nmc.org.uk/standards/guidance/raising-concerns-guidance-for-nurses-and-midwives

Nursing and Midwifery Council (NMC) (2015b) *The Code: Professional Standards of Practice and Behaviour for Nurses and Midwives:* London: NMC.

Public Concern at Work (2013) *Whistleblowing Commission Code of Practice*. Available at: http://www.pcaw.org.uk/files/PCaW_COP_FINAL.pdf

Whistleblower Interview Project (2012) *Margaret Haywood: How I Became a Whistleblower*. Available at: https://vimeo.com/53585810

Whitehead, B. and Barker, D. (2010) Does the risk of reprisal prevent nurses blowing the whistle on bad practice?, *Nursing Times*, 106(43): 12–15.

20 | What the research evidence says about being a newly qualified nurse

---

Overview

This chapter looks at the research base in order to provide a solid set of evidence for you to use in order to gain the best experience as a newly qualified nurse (NQN). The advice provided here is underpinned by the investigations into the most effective forms of preceptorship and how to encourage them conducted in our recent case study research project and our systematic review.

Introduction

As discussed in Chapter 3, evidence-based practice (EBP) is essential to provide the best care. It has been known for a long time that the period after qualifying is a difficult one for NQNs to travel through (Kramer, 1974). This chapter therefore outlines the evidence about the challenges and advantages of becoming an NQN and how you can use this to improve your own experiences.

Evidence from a systematic review and other studies

As part of a research project with an acute hospital, a National Health Service (NHS) Trust between 2010 and 2013, we conducted a systematic review of published primary research papers on preceptorship to support NQNs in the UK (Whitehead *et al.*, 2012; Whitehead *et al.*, 2013). This section uses evidence from this and from other research findings that have become available since the review; the findings are focused on here. However, should you wish to check the methods used to reach these results, the review and original papers are all publically available and can be located using the references. The most important findings and recommendations are described below.

What makes a supportive preceptorship programme

The most central result of the systematic review was that the majority of the papers reviewed had a research aim that was now proved: this was to find out if having a period of supported preceptorship was preferable to not having one or whether having a period of preceptorship was desirable at all. The conclusion from the review, perhaps unsurprisingly, was that in every case the researchers found that having some form of preceptorship after qualifying was preferable to not having any. This led to the recommendation for future research that researchers could dispense with identifying whether preceptorship was needed at all as this was undoubtedly proven. What should be focused on are ways to improve upon the good practice of providing NQNs with supported preceptorship.

The themes to focus on identified by the full systematic review were: 'Managerial Support Framework'; 'Recognition and Status of Role'; 'Protected Time for Preceptor and Preceptee'; 'Education Preparation of Preceptors'; 'Recruitment and Retention'; 'Competence of Preceptees'; 'Reflection and Critical Thinking in Action' (Whitehead *et al.*, 2012). All of these were important in ensuring that NQNs are properly supported during their initial transition from student to RN. The recommended actions based on these were as follows:

- A managerial support framework to be formed consisting of: a preceptorship lead for the hospital; clinical educators whose job it would be to support the clinical education of all staff including the NQNs in a ward or department; and a named preceptor for each NQN.
- The importance of the role and status of preceptors to be supported by the clinical educators and trust preceptorship lead.
- Preceptors and preceptees to have dedicated time allocated to the process. This to include a period of supernumerary time for preceptees.
- Each preceptor to undertake a course to prepare them for the role.
- Preceptorship is seen as essential by NQNs seeking their first job and the review indicated that retention was improved by preceptorship. Both of these things are important in a time of nursing shortages and therefore preceptorship is a worthwhile investment for employers.
- The confidence of NQNs to perform the tasks required at the point of registration was measurably lower than their actual ability to undertake them. Consequently, they should concentrate their efforts on improving their confidence rather than competency.
- It is necessary for NQNs to meet with peers in order to share and reflect upon their experiences. Otherwise, they become isolated and unfairly measure their performance against more experienced RNs.

As can be seen, the advice given above is mainly targeted at employers to provide them with an evidence-based guide to provide the best support for NQNs during preceptorship. However, as an NQN it is possible to use some of these recommendations to ensure that you have the best experience possible. First, it is worth checking that your employer has these actions in place. Second, some of the recommendations can be used directly by an NQN: you can develop a sense of feeling assured that you have completed a tough pre-registration course and should be confident in your abilities; and you can make sure that you discuss your experiences with peers who qualified at the same time as well as with more experienced nurses. This will help you to measure your level of competency against someone who is in a similar position rather than against someone with more experience. Even a few months at this stage in your professional life will make a huge difference. The reality shock (Kramer, 1974) of becoming an autonomous RN after being protected as a student remains, but can be mitigated by preceptorship support, confidence in your abilities and the peer support advised above. Dealing with reality shock is expanded upon in the next chapter.

A recent PhD thesis has indicated that the issue of incivility is a real problem to many NQNs (Halpin, 2015). It would be ideal for experienced nurses to treat NQNs with respect and understanding that they are learning the ropes. This would be expected if they could remember what it was like for them when they qualified but as often as not people's memories are nostalgic rather than accurate. This incivility is not usually at the level of deliberate bullying or unpleasantness but is rather usually perceived by the NQN as a lack of understanding and lack of welcome. Consequently, the NQN needs to become resilient if they are to survive their transition from student to RN. This is explored further in Chapter 24.

Evidence from the primary research report

The systematic review above was conducted as a basis for a case study research project. The case in question was all of the preceptorship activity in a medium-sized acute hospital (Whitehead, 2014; Whitehead *et al.*, 2016). The main findings in addition to those from the systematic review were that characteristics of a positive preceptorship are when the organization ensures that there is:

- individualization of preceptorship needs and ways to ensure successful preparation of students and NQNs
- support for NQNs in obtaining the right specialized skills for the specific job that they obtain in addition to the broad range of skills attained as part of their pre-registration education
- a culture of support in wards and departments supporting preceptees is encouraged and monitored
- peer support for preceptees and preceptors is provided
- confidence and resilience of preceptees is encouraged and supported
- technological support processes are included into preceptorship programmes to reduce isolation and encourage peer support.

These led to three headline recommendations for practice:

- Culture of support for preceptors and preceptees.
- Recognition of the preceptorship role within a governance framework including clinical educators.
- Individualized programme for each preceptee based on own needs and needs of their first area of employment.

These results are returned to in Chapter 25 as they lay the basis for the 'toolkit for transition' described in that chapter.

How can you use this evidence to improve your practice?

The findings indicated that the place of pre-registration practice and theory preparation made a difference to the speed in which the NQN made a successful transition to an accepted member of the RN team in their first workplace. That is not to say that you should necessarily try to find your first job with a local employer. It does mean that you should bear in mind that it will take longer to learn the ropes if your first job is at a workplace where you have never been on placement and even longer if it is with an overall employer that you have not been familiar with. This seems to be because knowing the routine, bureaucracy, expected conditions and organization of the clinical area makes it easier to get to grips with the more important aspects of professional transition such as being an autonomous decision maker and delegating activities safely. The advice to employers when providing preceptorship for NQNs is to give them more supernumerary time to settle in. Similarly, you should give yourself more time to feel part of the team when comparing yourself to peers who have had placements closer to their first RN post. In the scheme of things the amount of additional time needed is probably only a matter of a few weeks more. However, as the NQN going through this stage in your professional life, those few weeks will seem longer during the transition period than at any other time.

In a similar vein remember that students are prepared for a broad range of nursing skills and consequently many of the specific skills required for the jobs and specialties they find themselves in will need to be learned after qualification. It simply would not be practicable to learn every possible skill required for the wide range of posts that an NQN could find themselves in. Again as an NQN the best advice on this is to be prepared to learn the skills required for the job. Some of them will have been learned as a student, some of which will require you to revise them from the first year or may be fresh from your final placement. However, it is likely that some will be new to you and it is important that you either make your own arrangements to learn them yourself, such as the common medical conditions of patients in your care, or that you acknowledge to you preceptor that you need help in acquiring them, such as physical clinical skills which may not have been part of your pre-registration programme.

Conclusion

The most important thing from the evidence base to bear in mind is that the transition from student to RN is simply that: 'a transition'. Any feelings of anxiety that come with it will pass. The evidence from the systematic review and the primary research study above indicate that most nurses need between four and six months of support to start to feel like a member of the RN team. That said, when you are living it, those few months can be a long time and reality shock remains a concern for NQNs. Approaches to dealing with this are looked at in more detail in the next chapter.

References

Halpin, Y. (2015) *Newly Qualified Nurse Transition: Stress Experiences and Stress-mediating Factors – A Longitudinal Study*. PhD thesis. London Southbank University.

Kramer, M. (1974) *Reality Shock: Why Nurses Leave Nursing*. Saint Louis, MO: C. V. Mosby Co.

Whitehead, B. (2014) *Preceptorship Research Project Report*. Derby: Report, P. R. P. [Online]. Available at: https://drive.google.com/open?Id=0b80sguqmf6elsuvyzw1aagwyvwm

Whitehead, B., Holmes, D., Beddingham, E., Henshaw, L., Owen, P., Simmons, M. and Walker, C. (2012) *Preceptorship Programmes in the UK: A Systematic Literature Review*. [Online].

Available at: https://docs.google.com/file/d/0Bzzvt7Tfz8TKZEhNSkl5bmtyelk/edit?usp=sharing (accessed: 6 May 2016).

Whitehead, B., Owen, P., Holmes, D., Beddingham, E., Simmons, M., Henshaw, L., Barton, M. and Walker, C. (2013) Supporting newly qualified nurses in the UK: a systematic literature review, *Nurse Education Today*, 33(4): 370–377.

Whitehead, B., Owen, P., Henshaw, L., Beddingham, E. and Simmons, M. (2016) Supporting newly qualified nurse transition: a case study in a UK hospital, *Nurse Education Today*, 36: 58–63.

21 Dealing with reality shock

Overview

Reality shock is a phenomenon recognized in the literature about becoming a nurse. It is difficult to prepare you for this, but this chapter provides some advice and techniques to make the shock of the transition less of a burden.

Introduction

Kramer (1974) was one of the first nursing researchers to identify the concept of reality shock. It describes the feeling that newly qualified nurses (NQNs) get when they realize that the practicalities of being a registered nurse (RN) are different from those that they perhaps anticipated or, indeed, expected. Duchscher (2009) identified a similar phenomenon, more than 35 years later, and once again, more recent still, Whitehead *et al.* (2013) and Allan *et al.* (2016). Despite the introduction of a compulsory period of preceptorship (United Kingdom Central Council (UKCC) for Nursing, Midwifery and Health Visiting 1990), it remains an anxiety-provoking tsunami of emotions.

You will, however, progress through this state of uncertainty and feeling of being overwhelmed. Of course there will continue to be challenges throughout your career, but that initial period where you are perceived as newly qualified is a very condensed time of anxiety. You need to ensure that you maintain safe practice and do not compromise your care and eventually your time management will be easier, your ability to delegate and lead will be more effective, and you will feel more competent. These attributes and skills come with time as you embark on your new role as a staff nurse. In your training, you can simulate staff nurse activities and acknowledge the role models who inspire you, but you are not a staff nurse at that point and so do not have the pressures of accountability and the requirement to know and make decisions and manage and lead.

Meeting your preceptor

This is an important event and can help in establishing your needs, including your developmental aspirations as well as your concerns and anxieties in your new role. The Department of Health (DH) (2008) identified and suggested overwhelming support for the preceptorship model of support, stating that it will enable nurses to develop professionally and facilitate the transition from novice to expert. This journey has been identified by renowned theorists like Benner (1984) as an important journey not only for the nurse, but also for the patients they care for. It allows expertise to be developed through reflection and recognition of significant events. This recognition comes through acknowledging and recalling experiences. This is a supportive journey and may involve the support of a specific person or a group of individuals who may have aided your learning.

There are numerous models of support that nursing has adopted including mentoring, coaching and clinical supervision. One or all of these methods may be adopted to help support you through this transitional phase. Of course, this support does not only have to come from your preceptor; it can be other staff who offer it, or you might approach other staff to ask for the support. Coaching tends to involve the building of competency and results in motivation from doing the task or skill well as an end product (Bach and Ellis, 2011). Mentoring involves more role modelling and perhaps can be more closely linked with the preceptorship role than the former options. There may be a subtle difference in mentoring and coaching with mentoring being a greater interest in an individual's progress and personal growth rather than simply being proficient in a skill that tends to happen when a coaching style is adopted.

Undoubtedly, a number of methods may be utilized to aid you in achieving competency and confidence as well as effectiveness in your role. There are, of course, differences between mentoring in your pre-registration programme as the mentor in that case is a specified role which is acknowledged and associated with assessment of competency. The preceptor, who takes on a mentoring role, is not necessarily assessing you, but is supporting and guiding you. All qualified nurses have a duty to report poor or dangerous practice (NMC, 2015) and so assessment may be a discreet part of all qualified nurses, role but not in the same manner that is identified in the pre-registration education to support learning and assessment in practice.

What this suggests is that the relationship between preceptor and preceptee needs to be extensive and a true relationship based on trust and support. A further supportive model is clinical supervision.

Clinical supervision

Clinical supervision can be delivered by anyone; it does not specifically have to be your preceptor, a nurse in your environment or even a nurse at all. Bach and Ellis (2011) suggest that the preceptor, perhaps, incorporates a certain level of clinical supervision but a more robust form may be found by the NQN seeking out a supervisor of their own choice. Often the preceptors are allocated preceptees rather than the preceptee selecting a preceptor (Whitehead *et al.*, 2016). The fact that clinical supervision for qualified nurses is sparse (Bach and Ellis, 2011; Butterworth, 2007) may be partially due to the preceptor role, however, once preceptorship is complete, other supervision may be necessary for the welfare of the nurse. Clinical supervision is an opportunity to reflect with an unbiased party and may facilitate personal and professional growth through the activity of reflective discussion. Thomas (2006) identifies that the only real factor to consider is that the supervisor should be someone with greater experience so that their support can perhaps be more directive and, more importantly, correct.

The supervision should be available at times of need so you gain some responsiveness from them. This may be a challenge when many practitioners have time limitation. The trust surrounding negotiation of time and ascertaining realistic support is essential.

Peer support

Other ways of easing transition to a NQN is to gain peer support (Whitehead *et al.*, 2013). Just as you found peer support invaluable in your transition to student nurse, entering your pre-registration programme, peer support in your transition to qualified nurse can also be equally beneficial. Forming groups with other NQNs can achieve the sharing and other associated, supportive benefits that can make you feel less isolated and alone. It can give that added sense of being cared for and the ability to share concerns in that caring environment (Brock and Brown, 2016). It can also be reassuring that others are undergoing similar concerns and experiences. There is always the chance that there may be some element of panic as one member can bring up an issue that others have not considered and then leading to a sense of mass anxiety, but the advantages should far outweigh the potential drawbacks.

Case study 21.1: Leanne

Leanne was feeling anxious as she had experienced three very difficult days on the ward. This was her third week and she was expecting it to get easier day by day, not more difficult. She really was starting to question her suitability and the more threats and challenges that were presented, the more panicked she began to feel. She was worried she was going to make a big mistake. Her preceptor reassured her that this was ok and that everyone had off days but it felt like more than an 'off' day. She decided to contact some of her fellow NQNs. She arranged a catch up, away from work. Fifteen attended. Initially, everyone was suggesting it was all great. Her fears started to become a reality until one nurse spoke up and said, actually, hers was not great and she was having a difficult time. Soon they started sharing experiences in a more meaningful way and progressed to problem solving and sharing of ideas. They agreed that it had been an extremely positive gathering and decided that they would do it on a regular basis. They exchanged contact details so that they could call on one another if there were significant difficulties or wanted advice or a sounding board.

Reflection

- How constructive do you think this was?
- Could you consider sharing concerns with your peers?

Conclusion

Often sharing problems can be cathartic in itself. Also, problem solving as a collective can be an effective way of dealing with difficult situations. Sometimes we are too close to the issue to see a route or a solution. What is important is that experiencing a period of transitional support can help ease anxiety, confidence and job satisfaction (Edwards *et al.*, 2015), and as a byproduct it may help the health organization you work for retain staff (Whitehead *et al.*, 2013). If a staff nurse stays in their post, it generally indicates they may be satisfied, fulfilled and valued. The support you receive will have an impact on whether you can feel this way, even if not at the start of your time in the post when you are still adjusting to the transition. When attaining your first newly qualified post, take the opportunity to question the support available, and question the preceptorship provision, ensuring it is robust and well organized. Although one cannot be certain of this, asking questions may be a good way of ascertaining this.

Competency and confidence come with experience and engagement in learning. Learning can be achieved in a number of ways and you need to find the most effective way to suit your needs. Sharing your concerns and anxieties can help others identify your needs and can allow them to provide individualized, responsive, support. This is essential as you ease your way through the transition from student nurse to newly qualified staff nurse to experienced practitioner.

References

Allan, H., Magnusson, C., Evans, K., Ball, E., Westwood, S., Curtis, K., Horton, K. and Johnson, M. (2016) Delegation and supervision of healthcare assistants' work in the daily management of uncertainty and the unexpected in clinical practice: invisible learning among newly qualified nurses, *Nursing Inquiry*, 23(4): 377–385.

Bach, S. and Ellis, P. (2011) *Leadership, Management and Team Working in Nursing*. London: Learning Matters/Sage.

Benner, P. (1984) *From Novice to Expert: Excellence and Power in Clinical Nursing Practice*. Menlo Park, CA: Addison-Wesley Publishing Company.

Brock, M. and Brown, M. (2016) Support for the practitioner, in Brown, M., *Palliative Care for Nursing and Healthcare*. London: Sage.

Butterworth, T., Bell, L., Jackson, C. and Majda, P. (2007) Wicked spell or magic bullet? A review of the clinical supervision literature 2001–2007, *Nurse Education Today*, 28(3): 264–272.

Department of Health (DH) (2008) *End of Life Care Strategy*. London: DH.

Duchscher, J. E. (2009) Transition shock theory: the initial stage of role adaptation for newly qualified nurses, *Journal of Advanced Nursing*, 65(5): 1103–1113.

Edwards, D., Hawker, C., Carrier, J. and Rees, C. (2015) A systematic review of the effectiveness of strategies and interventions to improve the transition from student to qualified nurse, *International Journal of Nursing Studies*, 52(7): 1254–1268.

Kramer, M. (1974) *Reality Shock: Why Nurses Leave Nursing*. St Louis, MO: C. V. Mosby.

Thomas, J. (2006) *Survival Guide for Ward Managers, Sisters and Charge Nurses*. London: Churchill Livingstone Elsevier.

United Kingdom Central Council (UKCC) for Nursing, Midwifery and Health Visiting (1990) *The Report of the Post-registration Education and Practice Project*. London: UKCC.

Whitehead, B., Owen, P., Holmes, D., Beddingham, E., Simmons, M., Henshaw, L., Barton, M. and Walker, C. (2013) Supporting newly qualified nurses in the UK: a systematic literature review, *Nurse Education Today*, 33(4): 370–377.

Whitehead, B., Owen, P., Henshaw, L., Beddingham, E. and Simmons, M. (2016) Supporting newly qualified nurse transition: a case study in a UK hospital, *Nurse Education Today*, 36: 58–63.

22 Making the most of preceptorship

Overview

As a newly qualified nurse (NQN), you will have a named preceptor allocated to you. The evidence shows that preceptorship is effective as a way of supporting NQNs but that the local interpretation of preceptorship does vary. You will need to be prepared therefore to ensure that you gain meaningful preceptorship. This chapter helps you consider what preceptorship is and how to make the most of it.

Introduction

Since 1990 the nursing regulator, the NMC, has advised that all NQNs should have a period of support called preceptorship (United Kingdom Central Council (UKCC) for Nursing, Midwifery and Health Visiting, 1990; Nursing and Midwifery Council (NMC), 2006). This has not yet been made into an NMC professional requirement but NHS employers have been required to follow the Department of Health (DH) (2010) Preceptorship Framework for many years. Consequently, if your first job is with a National Health Service (NHS) employer, then you should be guaranteed to be provided with a period of preceptorship and many private and voluntary sector employers also do this.

What is preceptorship?

In the context of nursing in the UK, preceptorship has a specific professional definition: 'the process through which existing nurses and midwives provide support to newly qualified nurses and midwives' (NMC, 2008: 46). The NMC stipulate that:

Preceptorship is about providing support and guidance enabling 'new registrants' to make the transition from student to accountable practitioner to:

practise in accordance with the NMC code of professional conduct: standards for conduct, performance and ethics;

develop confidence in their competence as a nurse, midwife or specialist community public health nurse;

To facilitate this the 'new registrant' should have:

learning time protected in their first year of qualified practice; and

have access to a preceptor with whom regular meetings are held.

NMC (2006: 1)

Preceptorship is therefore a technical term for the period of support for the NQN from another more experienced nurse. The regulator goes on to explain that preceptors should have at least one year's experience and have a teaching qualification such as a mentor course.

As mentioned in the introduction, the most up-to-date definition for the NHS encompasses nurses and allied health professions and is defined by the DH as:

> A period of structured transition for the newly registered practitioner during which he or she will be supported by a preceptor, to develop their confidence as an autonomous professional, refine skills, values and behaviours and to continue on their journey of life-long learning.
>
> DH (2010: 11)

It is worth picking this definition apart as there are a series of important themes in it that are supported by the research evidence outlined in Chapter 20. It makes it clear that the point of the support of the preceptor within the employer's structured preceptorship programme is to:

1. develop the confidence of the NQN rather than to test and retrain them
2. refine the NQN's existing skills for the particular clinical area they are in
3. build upon their existing values and behaviours as a registered nurse (RN)
4. continue their journey of lifelong learning rather than qualification being an end of education for a fully formed RN.

Preceptorship is intended to be a supportive period following registration rather than an extension of your pre-registration course. Consequently, your preceptor should not be seen as another NMC mentor. As explained in previous chapters, the mentor's purpose is to teach and assess the student on their placement. The most important professional purpose of this relationship is to ensure that the student is worthy of joining the register. The preceptor's purpose cannot be to reassess the NQN as they have already undergone this process as a student and been signed off by mentors throughout their course. The preceptor's purpose is to support the NQN through the reality shock of transition from protected student to autonomous RN. Of course, NQNs and all other employees are subject to assessment of their competency throughout their career. However, the appropriate person to enforce this assessment is their line manager rather than their preceptor.

Supported preceptorship has been developed over the years and now is often overseen by a preceptorship lead within the employing organization and this is encouraged by the DH (2010). The preceptorship leads also often learn and share best practice with national and regional preceptorship and clinical educator networks such as the UK Clinical Nurse Educator Network (Whitehead and Allibone, 2016). Nevertheless, the nature and quality of preceptorship varies from employer to employer.

Find out about local preceptorship support

One of the most important questions to ask at an interview, and to check with current NQN employees if possible, is: what preceptorship package is available? Your professional life will be off to a great start if your first post is well supported through the transition from student to RN. Consequently, as preceptorship support can vary widely from employer to employer and even between departments within one entity, it is worth checking before you accept a post what level of support is likely to be available. It is also worth considering that NQNs often change jobs soon after starting if the post turns out not to be the right one for them. As nursing are in short supply, it is relatively straightforward in most circumstances to do this, and therefore if the promise of preceptorship support is not honoured, you should not feel obliged to remain in post longer than your notice period allows. This may sound disloyal but a contract of employment requires commitment from both sides. If the employer is not prepared to support you through this vulnerable stage in your development, then it is worth finding one who will.

Case study 22.1 illustrates a dilemma you might face.

Case study 22.1: Preceptorship support

You have started work as an NQN in an outpatients department (OPD). On starting work at the hospital you and the other NQNs are provided with an induction programme consisting of face-to-face and online mandatory training such as manual handling and infection control. In addition to the workplace health and safety, you are introduced to the trust's preceptorship lead, Kath. She provides you with a preceptorship handbook that explains all of the local preceptorship support procedures and a series of monthly workshops where you can meet with other preceptees and the trust preceptorship team. Kath also informs you of the name of the more experienced RN at the outpatients who will be your preceptor. This all sounds exciting and when you arrive at work the next day you are greeted by your preceptor Eve. She welcomes you to the OPD and shows you around. There seems like a lot to learn as you have never had an OPD as a placement. The next day arrives and you are expecting to be working with Eve again. However, Eve has been moved to another department due to staff shortages. The other nurses are really busy and you are not sure of the routine yet and they all seem annoyed that you do not know what to do. One of them says to an other: 'Oh no we have another one of these useless NQNs. Don't they teach them anything in university anymore? We just used to get on with it.'

Reflection

1. Consider how this would make you feel.
2. Is there any justification in them saying this?
3. What would you do under these circumstances?

In this case, the NQN had found one of the majority of employers that provides a structured and evidence-based preceptorship programme with a named preceptor and a trust-wide programme. What appears to be missing in this case is the local culture of support. In our research, preceptees reported that the most important element of preceptorship was that the ward, department or community nursing team were all aware of the need to give the NQN time to learn the ropes in the workplace and to provide them with support and understanding during their period of transition (Whitehead *et al.*, 2016). This is the final and perhaps most important thing to be aware of when finding out about the local preceptorship support. If the team at the workplace are understanding and empathetic towards the needs of NQNs, then it is likely that everything else will fall into place.

How to ensure that you have a meaningful preceptorship

Once you have checked that the workplace has an overall organizational preceptorship programme, that the workplace has a team which will provide a community of support, and that you will be allocated a named preceptor, then you are half way there to ensuring that you have a meaningful preceptorship. However, whether these things are available or not, there are some steps that you can take in order to ensure the best experience practicable.

1. Find the time to meet regularly with your preceptor. It is often difficult in a busy workplace to find the time to make sure that things are progressing as they should. Nevertheless, at this stage in your career you need to discuss your progress and to make sure that you understand your role with your preceptor on a regular basis. In our research, preceptors commented that they did not want to ask to meet their preceptees formally unless the preceptee requested it. This was because they thought that the preceptee would believe they were checking up on them and that they were not satisfied with their performance. However, if the preceptee asked for a discussion they would find the time to do it.
2. Make sure that if the employer has organized times to meet with other preceptees that you take advantage of these. There are several different approaches to these peer support groups. Some employers have regular study days for NQNs on a variety of subjects. Some have action learning sets or other forms of peer supervision sessions. Whatever the structure you should try to ensure that you take the time to attend these as it is an invaluable way of reassuring yourself that you are progressing at a reasonable rate compared to your NQN colleagues.
3. Take advantage of any learning experience. Remember, that as an NQN you may have completed your pre-registration studies but this is just the start of your lifelong learning journey. During your course you were studying to be an RN. Now you are learning to be a functional nurse in the speciality that you have selected to work on. Learning experiences such as drug administration, multidisciplinary team (MDT) meetings, observing procedures as well as private study of the issues generated by practice will all help you to become a proficient and finally an expert nurse in this aspect of nursing practice.
4. Smile. You have made it. You are an RN with a licence to care for patients who need your expertise and compassion. Go out there and make a difference!

Conclusion

A lot of thought, research and planning has gone into preparing the preceptorship programmes around the country to support NQNs like yourself. Things can and do go wrong but for the majority of NQNs this is an exciting as well as stressful time that is rightly supported by a team of professionals. Remember that you have succeeded in completing a tough pre-registration programme and have joined the nursing register that will enable you to practise in the profession of your choice: nursing. Through your studies, hard work and dedication you are in a privileged position, at the beginning of a professional career, with emotional and vocational rewards that the majority of people can only dream of.

References

Department of Health (DH) (2010) *Preceptorship Framework for Newly Registered Nurses, Midwives and Allied Health Professionals.* London: DH.

Nursing and Midwifery Council (NMC) (2006) *Preceptorship Guidelines: NMC Circular 21/2006.* London: NMC. Available at: https://www.nmc.org.uk/globalassets/sitedocuments/circulars/2006circulars/nmc-circular-21_2006.pdf

Nursing and Midwifery Council (NMC) (2008) *Standards to Support Learning and Assessment in Practice.* London: NMC.

United Kingdom Central Council (UKCC) for Nursing, Midwifery and Health Visiting (1990) *The Report of the Post-registration Education and Practice Project.* London: UKCC.

Whitehead, B. and Allibone, L. (2016) *Clinical Nurse Educator Network UK.* Available at: www.derby.ac.uk/CNEnet (accessed: 8 October 2016).

Whitehead, B., Owen, P., Henshaw, L., Beddingham, E. and Simmons, M. (2016) Supporting newly qualified nurse transition: a case study in a UK hospital, *Nurse Education Today*, 36: 58–63.

23 **Why you should be confident**

Overview

Confidence is an important part in the newly qualified nurse's (NQN) delivery of patient care. It can be knocked by the shock of the reality of becoming an autonomous registrant. This chapter examines the reasons for lack of confidence and provides advice on building up your confidence to the appropriate level. In addition, as an NQN you must know your own limitations and have the assertiveness to be able to admit when you are at the edge of your abilities. Both of these issues are dealt with in this chapter.

Introduction

You have trained to be a generalist and you will be expected to be a specialist on whatever job you start off at. This will lead you to go from competent senior student to novice registered nurse in the particular speciality you find yourself (Benner, 1984). As a sweeping generalization, experienced nurses have probably always considered that the current generation of NQNs are less competent and not as well trained as they were. This was the central argument of the changes made to nurse education at the end of the twentieth century (Department of Health (DH), 1999; United Kingdom Central Council (UKCC) for Nursing, 1999) and this attitude was a feature of a ground-breaking and often cited study of a London teaching hospital in the 1950s (Menzies, 1960). However, the reality is that nurses join the profession now for similar reasons to the ones given throughout history (Crick *et al.*, 2014) and the education programmes are designed by experienced RNs. In addition, students are taught and assessed by RNs in theory and practice. Our research indicated that NQNs have the competency to do their job but they lack the confidence in their own ability and partly as a consequence other staff lack confidence in them (Whitehead *et al.*, 2013; Whitehead *et al.*, 2016). The difficulty appears to be that pre-registration programmes cannot hope to prepare nurses for every possible job that they may find themselves in. Consequently, there is likely to be a period of time after qualifying when the NQN is likely to have a temporary lack of confidence. This chapter examines this and ways of alleviating it.

Reasons for this temporary lack of confidence

As indicated above, it is hardly surprising that NQNs do not have the full range of skills for the specific speciality in their first post. What they will have are the necessary professional building blocks of a body of nursing knowledge and the general range of fundamental and RN level skills required by nurses across the board. These will certainly include the Essential Skills Clusters listed by the Nursing and Midwifery Council (NMC) (2010). Consequently, within the limits of your competency, there is every rational reason to be confident in your abilities.

The reported lack of confidence comes in part from what Kramer described as reality shock and later Duchscher described as transition shock (Kramer, 1974; Duchscher, 2009). This is the shock of understanding what it is like to be an autonomous qualified nurse rather than a protected student. With this new responsibility comes the realization that there is a lot to learn in your new environment and in your new profession. This may appear obvious but what is not so obvious to the NQN is that the most essential parts of this vast sphere of knowledge and skills have been proven repeatedly to be possible to learn within the first few months of qualifying but importantly simply cannot be embedded properly until you have the title of RN. Consequently, it is important to prepare yourself as much as possible for the role while you are a student but also to realize that you cannot live the experience of being an RN until you are one.

Various factors including reality shock, a daunting realization of the amount to learn, some less than civil words from co-workers and the need to learn the ropes in a new working environment are likely to be the cause for a lack of confidence in many NQNs immediately after qualification. Unfortunately, the evidence indicates that this feeling does not entirely dissipate for a few months after qualifying. However, it may be heartening to hear that the majority of NQNs report that as they gain competency and proficiency in the various tasks that seemed so daunting at first, they start to feel more confident in their overall abilities to provide the holistic care to their patients.

Advice on building up your confidence

Nilsson *et al.* (2005) have identified that confidence can be engendered in the workplace by organizational efforts to provide networks similar to those indicated by our preceptorship research (Whitehead *et al.*, 2016). It may be that you have arrived in an enlightened working environment of this kind that will acknowledge that NQNs should be expected to lack confidence at first and consequently have built a community of support and organizational elements, such as a network of peer support, to help you to quickly raise your self-confidence. This will also encourage others to have confidence in your abilities as they develop. However, even though there are national frameworks to encourage organizations to do this, it may not be the reality you have to deal with. In either case you can improve your own self-confidence by taking your own actions.

Reflection

1. Look back over your work as a student to remind yourself of the educational and professional journey that you have travelled in a few short years and try to imagine how much you will learn in the next few years as an RN.

2. Think back over your nurse education and consider whether your course taught any techniques for confidence building, stress management and learning skills?
3. Go back to any that you found helpful and practise them with regard to your experiences as an RN.

As indicated in the reflection exercises, there are many techniques for confidence building. A common method is to assess your current position with a view to goal or objective setting in order to see where you are now and how to get from here to where you want to be. This can be through a SWOT (strengths, weaknesses, opportunities and threats) analysis as described below.

	Helpful to achieving the objective	**Harmful** to achieving the objective
Internal origin	*Strengths*	*Weaknesses*
External origin	*Opportunities*	*Threats*

In the context of improving self-confidence and awareness of your abilities, this would likely be a list of the *strengths* you have gathered by study and clinical practice as a student; *weaknesses* may be the gaps that you perceive in your knowledge and skills in relation to the speciality of care in your new workplace; *opportunities* are likely to be the chances to use your skills and knowledge to care for patients and to be exposed to new learning experiences within a community of supportive staff; and finally *threats* could be the potential for incivility from staff who have forgotten what it was like to be an NQN.

When all of this is committed to paper, it can often seem more manageable as it then becomes a list of experiences and actions to complete rather than something unachievable.

Know your limits

The evidence indicates that NQNs should be more confident than they are because, when competency is measured objectively against the NQN's perception of their ability, they usually assess themselves lower than they deserve (Holland *et al.*, 2010). However, there is the possibility of overdoing this and being confident beyond your current ability. The most important advice is to know your limits and not go beyond them. If you find yourself in a situation where you feel that you are out of your depth, you should acknowledge this to both yourself and your preceptor. Remember you are just starting out on your learning journey and everyone will progress at different rates with separate parts of the overall role. If there are aspects of the job that you are finding trickier to get to grips with than you or your preceptor expected, this is not something to hide. It is to be expected and recognizing it can enable you to concentrate on this part of the role in order to master it.

Conclusion

Often, for a few months, NQNs will feel less confident of their ability to do the job than they were as a student. This is to be expected for the reasons indicated above. However, you have good reason to feel self-confident, while knowing your limits, and your confidence will help others feel confident in your ability and to trust you to be a valuable member of the team and someone who will provide good quality care to patients. As Christopher Robin said: 'Always remember you are braver than you believe, stronger than you seem, and smarter than you think.'

References

Benner, P. E. (1984) *From Novice to Expert: Excellence and Power in Clinical Nursing Practice.* Menlo Park, CA: Addison-Wesley Publishing Company, Nursing Division.

Crick, P., Perkinton, L. and Davies, F. (2014) Why do student nurses want to be nurses?, *Nursing Times*, 110(5): 12–15.

Department of Health (DH) (1999) *Making a Difference: Strengthening the Nursing, Midwifery and Health Visiting Contribution to Health and Healthcare; Summary.* London: DH.

Duchscher, J. E. (2009) Transition shock: the initial stage of role adaptation for newly graduated registered nurses, *Journal of Advanced Nursing*, 65(5): 1103–1113.

Holland, K., Roxburgh, M., Johnson, M., Topping, K., Watson, R., Lauder, W. and Porter, M. (2010) Fitness for practice in nursing and midwifery education in Scotland, United Kingdom, *Journal of Clinical Nursing*, 19(3/4): 461–469.

Kramer, M. (1974) *Reality Shock: Why Nurses leave Nursing.* Saint Louis, MO: C. V. Mosby Co.

Menzies, I. E. P. (1960) A case study in the functioning of social systems as a defence against anxiety: a report on a study of the nursing service of a general hospital, *Human Relations*, 13(2): 95–121.

Nilsson, K., Hertting, A., Petterson, I.-L. and Theorell, T. (2005) Pride and confidence at work: potential predictors of occupational health in a hospital setting, *BMC Public Health*, 5: 92.

Nursing and Midwifery Council (NMC) (2010) *Standards for Pre-Registration Nursing Education*. London: NMC.

United Kingdom Central Council (UKCC) for Nursing, Midwifery and Health Visiting (1999) *Fitness for Practice: The UKCC Commission for Nursing and Midwifery Education*. London: UKCC.

Whitehead, B., Owen, P., Holmes, D., Beddingham, E., Simmons, M., Henshaw, L., Barton, M. and Walker, C. (2013) Supporting newly qualified nurses in the UK: a systematic literature review, *Nurse Education Today*, 33(4): 370–377.

Whitehead, B., Owen, P., Henshaw, L., Beddingham, E. and Simmons, M. (2016) Supporting newly qualified nurse transition: a case study in a UK hospital, *Nurse Education Today*, 36(1): 58–63.

24 How to be resilient

Overview

Resilience is necessary for all professionals. However, as a newly qualified nurse (NQN) you are at a particularly vulnerable stage in your career, and so you need to have resilience and self-belief that will enable you to make it through this part of your journey. It goes without saying that organizations and fellow nurses should support you during your period of readjustment. Nevertheless, not every encounter will be a positive one. This chapter examines methods of achieving and retaining resilience in order to weather the storms that will invariably come into all RNs' lives.

Introduction

The consistent theme surrounding resilience is said to be the 'bouncing back', coping consistently in adverse situations (Hart *et al.*, 2014). One may question, however, whether this is sustainable without considering unburdening and recognizing one's own emotional distress. Mindfulness, which can help you do this, is currently receiving significant recognition surrounding its importance in alleviating stress and depression (Department of Health (DH), 2012; Hofmann *et al.*, 2010; Grossman *et al.*, 2004, Fjorback *et al.*, 2011; Merkes, 2010; Baer, 2003) and some studies relating to this are explored in the next section.

The Royal College of Nursing (2013) identified that, in a climate of understaffing and pressure, to be more financially efficient can threaten our ability to be caring and compassionate to ourselves. However, to be aware of, not only your patients' distress, but also how that distress is affecting you as a professional, can help to aid and maintain health and well-being. This chapter helps you to understand and identify the pressures you may face but, more importantly, how you may overcome these and maintain your own health and well-being and that of your fellow colleagues.

Compassion and self-awareness

Being critical of oneself and focusing on our mistakes may dominate us as NQNs. If you look back at Chapter 21, Case study 21.1 illustrates this. Leanne felt that she was unable to deal with the realities of being a staff nurse; she could not deal with the fact that she was not completely confident or competent. Of greater significance for her well-being, she did not appear to acknowledge to herself that she was safe, which, one may argue, is the most important quality an NQN can possess. In the long term this can cause significant harm; for example, burnout (Irving, 2009) as we are failing to be compassionate and forgiving of ourselves when things may not go to plan or meet our high standards. Brock and Brown (2016) have suggested that nurses often fail to be kind to themselves, and Gilbert (2009) has identified a strong link between compassion to oneself and compassion to others. It may be that, as our self-compassion diminishes, so too might the compassion for others. This will obviously have a detrimental impact on patient care.

Interventions

Many organizations have been employing mindfulness programmes in the hope to increase self-compassion within the workforce and thus increasing the resilience towards the stressful situations and experiences they may be facing and have to face in the future (Shonin *et al.*, 2014). The outcomes of these types of intervention have been determined beneficial in a holistic manner (Klatt and Fish, 2016). Perhaps by being forgiving of ourselves, we can reduce the self-punishment and allow greater resilience. Facing our failures, acknowledging their presence, building on, learning and using our experiences for something greater may enhance our practice, our patient care but also our own well-being.

Nursing may be seen as a demanding profession, emotionally, psychologically, physically, socially and even one may argue spiritually at times, forcing us to question our belief. We tend to engage with our patients in a very personal and intimate way that is a privilege but, when patients relay their innermost fears and confide their anxieties, then, we have to be able to manage their fears but also perhaps address our own. Dealing with breaking bad news to a patient and responding to their distress, their questions, their emotional response can be challenging but it can make this much worse if we have unrealistic expectations of how we should or could have dealt with the situation. We always want to be excellent in practice and the reality is that this might not always happen. Situations may be misjudged, there may be difficulty in answering questions, or we may feel unable to deal with the situation altogether, and these feelings and uncertainties, if left, may lead to our suffering. It is likely that resilience will not be sustained without acknowledgement of these challenges.

Scarf *et al.* (2013) undertook a mindfulness-based stress reduction intervention for midwives. They recognized that healthcare practitioners are faced with increasingly complex and stressful situations and mindfulness-based intervention can help alleviate the negative impact this may have on the professional long term, thereby increasing the opportunity for employing staff with the capacity to maintain their practice, increase well-being, increase resilience and reduce sickness and absence through work-related stress in the long term. Gauthier (2015), again, examined the potential benefits of mindfulness interventions. This was a paediatric intensive care unit. Once again, acknowledging the greater potential for stress with little chance for self-care, nurses have a predisposition to stress and burnout. They utilized mindfulness meditation resulting in a significant decrease in burnout and stress. Although they did not determine an increase in self-compassion and mindfulness, a relationship was seen between high stress and low self-compassion and mindfulness.

Mindfulness

Mindfulness, self-kindness and common humanity have been identified by Neff (2011; Neff and Pommier, 2012) as components of self-compassion. Lack of acknowledgment or attention to our needs can lead us to focus on our deficits and our faults, and result in withdrawal. Brock and Brown (2016) identified that mindfulness, recognizing our own hurt, fears, faults and distress is not a failure but one that is needed for well-being, but it requires practice and courage. Acknowledging we have faults may be difficult to digest because, in the pursuit of our daily role as a staff nurse, we can perceive that the expertise that is all around us is faultless. One may question whether this is realistic. We are human and may make unwise choices at times. As long as we are safe in our practice and recognize our own limitations and knowledge deficits, the faults should not be significant. A missed diagnosis can occur no matter what the profession, but, as long as you conducted accurate assessments and acted on them appropriately then there should be no self-reproach.

Case study 24.1: Julie

Julie worked in the community and had a significant caseload of patients, three of which were approaching the end of their lives. She had seen a significant number of patients over the last year in this situation and was continually reflecting on the quality of death she managed to achieve for all her patients. She could not get the situations as she wanted. Issues like failure to identify end of life, inability to get adequate resources in place, difficulties attaining adequate pain control and unresolvable family dynamics had been some of the difficulties. Rather than focus on what she had achieved and learning from those situations, Julie ruminated and was now at the point that she felt this caseload was overwhelming. The other difficulty was that she did not want to appear weak and so did not ask for help or discuss her anxieties.

Reflection

- In the long term, how do you think this will affect Julie?
- How could this have an impact on patient care?
- How could her colleagues help?

Julie is suffering, she is adopting very little, if any, compassion for herself and she is in danger of failing to cope with her caseload of patients. Julie has left her anxieties and distressing experiences unresolved for too long and now may need significant supervision. Her health and well-being is at substantial risk. This is a situation that can and should be avoided. As a nurse, facing these emotional challenges and demands, there are many ways to help you to cope with the challenges you may be faced with. Some strategies that may be helpful include ensuring you reflect on your practice and experiences, access supervision to discuss cases to ensure you have the ability to continue to provide the level of care you want to achieve but, in addition, to ensure you maintain your health and well-being.

There are a variety of exercises and methods that may be adopted to help you deal with distress and what may be termed 'the troubled self'. Brock and Brown (2016) have suggested a number of these that may help you to understand your distress but also help you to recover.

Conclusion

Self-compassion and resilience are paramount for health and social care professionals working in today's and tomorrow's healthcare environment. We are facing ever-increasing challenges relating to patient throughput, greater clinical demands, and the requirement for greater expertise in health and social care provision. This can all add to the challenges we currently face as a professional. Taking care of ourselves is vital in order to be able to take care of our colleagues, patients and families. We also have our own families and loved ones to care about, therefore being mindful in our role and compassionate to ourselves is vital.

References

Baer, R. A. (2003) Mindfulness training as a clinical intervention: a conceptual and empirical review, *Clinical Psychology*, 10(2): 125–143.

Brock, M. and Brown, M. (2016) Support for the practitioner, in Brown, M., *Palliative Care for Nursing and Healthcare*. London, Sage.

Department of Health (DH) (2012) *Compassion in Practice: Nursing, Midwifery and Care Staff – Our Vision and Strategy*. London: DH.

Fjorback, L., Arendt, M., Ornbol, E., Fink, P. and Walach, H. (2011) Mindfulness-based stress reduction and mindfulness-based cognitive therapy: a systematic review of randomised controlled trials, *Acta Psychiatrica Scandinavica*, 124(2): 102–109.

Gauthier, T. (2015) An on-the-job mindfulness-based intervention for pediatric ICU nurses: a pilot, *Journal of Pediatric Nursing*, 30(2): 402–409.

Gilbert, P. (2009). *The Compassionate Mind: A New Approach to Facing the Challenges of Life*. London: Constable Robinson.

Grossman, P., Niemann, L., Schmidt, S. and Walach, H. (2004) Mindfulness-based stress reduction and health benefits: a meta-analysis, *Journal of Psychosomatic Research*, 57(1): 35–43.

Hart, P., Brannan, J. D. and De Chesnay, M. (2014) Resilience in nurses: an integrative review, *Journal of Nursing Management*, 22(6): 720–734.

Hofmann, S. G., Sawyer, A. T. and Witt, A. A. (2010) The effect of mindfulness-based therapy on anxiety and depression: a meta-analytic review, *Journal of Consulting and Clinical Psychology*, 78(2): 169–183.

Irving, J. A., Dobkin, P. L. and Park, J. (2009) Cultivating mindfulness in health care professionals: a review of empirical studies of mindfulness-based stress reduction, *Complementary Therapies in Clinical Practice*, 15(2): 61–66.

Klatt, M. D., Wise, E. and Fish, M. (2016) Mindfulness and work-related well-being, in Shonin, E., Van Gordon, W. and Griffiths, M. D. (eds) *Mindfulness and Buddist-derived Approaches in Mental Health and Addiction.* New York: Springer.

Merkes, M. (2010) Mindfulness-based stress reduction for people with chronic diseases, *Australian Journal of Primary Health,* 16(3): 200–210.

Neff, K. D. (2011) *Self-compassion.* New York: William Morrow.

Neff, K. D. and Pommier, E. (2012) The relationship between self-compassion and other-focused concern among college undergraduates, community adults, and practicing meditators, *Self and Identity,* 12(2): 160–176.

Royal College of Nursing (2013) *Mid Staffordshire NHS Foundation Trust Public Inquiry Report: Response of the Royal College of Nursing.* London: The Stationery Office.

Scarf, V., Foureur, M., Crisp, J., Burton, G. and Yu, N. (2013) Efficacy of mindfulness based stress reduction (MBSR) on the sense of wellbeing of healthcare staff: a pilot study, *Women and Birth,* 26(17): 1–21.

Shonin, E., Van Gordon, W., Dunn, T. J., Singh, N. N. and Griffiths, M. D. (2014) Meditation awareness training (MAT) for work-related wellbeing and job performance: a randomized controlled trial, *International Journal of Mental Health and Addiction,* 12(6): 806–823.

25 Toolkit for transition

Introduction

This final chapter examines the evidence-based preceptorship toolkit that was generated by our research. They are shown in four figures that are tools or frameworks that can be followed to help create a successful system of support. These can be used to reflect upon the previous chapters, especially those relating to starting successfully as a registered nurse (RN). The final figure (Figure 25.5) in this chapter suggests a framework for measuring the progress of your transition from student to RN.

Explore the toolkit for transition

The toolkit that has been developed is intended to provide a framework to assist employers of newly qualified nurses (NQNs) to devise the best possible system of support. This will also help NQNs to understand the structures of support that are, or could be, available to them through this transition period. The findings of the research (Whitehead *et al.*, 2016) indicate that there are three levels required to optimize the support required by NQNs. The levels are:

1. The organizational support structure. This is the overall framework of support provided by the NHS trust or other healthcare employer for all of its NQNs.
2. The 'culture of support' within each of the areas (ward, department, community team, etc.) where the NQN begins their career.
3. The way in which individual one-to-one preceptorship is facilitated and ensured.

Consequently, this is a tool to support these three levels throughout the organization.

The research resulting from the project described above had, as its primary aim, the production of a toolkit to support employers in developing the best possible preceptorship programme for NQNs. The findings of the research generated a list of recommendations (Whitehead *et al.*, 2016). These findings and recommendations for practice fed into the production of the preceptorship support toolkit. There are four sections to the toolkit. Each section provides a mechanism for improving the preceptorship programme in different aspects of the preceptorship process. These are:

- Organizational support (Figure 25.1)
- Managerial support (Figure 25.2)

- Supernumerary time (Figure 25.3)
- Local culture of support (Figure 25.4)

The descriptions of each component of the toolkit and how to use them in practice follow.

The organizational support tool

In order to obtain the best outcome, the preceptorship lead for the organization can use the tool to implement or facilitate the themes listed in Figure 25.1. The preceptorship lead can also continuously monitor their organization to ensure that the themes are being addressed. For each theme the tool has a 'slider' to indicate the elements or activities required to provide the optimum conditions for transition supported by preceptorship. The activities are listed under each numbered theme heading as activity a, b, c, and so on.

The managerial support framework

The managerial support framework describes a structure supported by the evidence to ensure that the aspects of the toolkit are implemented and therefore that support is provided for NQNs undergoing preceptorship. It is a three-level hierarchy: preceptorship lead; ward-based preceptorship support facilitator; and preceptors. Each level should be provided with a number of hours out of their clinical role to undertake the preceptorship tasks and each should be required to support and monitor the level below them to ensure that the preceptees receive the preceptorship required. This is illustrated in Figure 25.2.

This research indicated that a structure of managerial support is required to ensure that the steps agreed at organizational level are implemented. It was found that it is necessary to have managers, supervisors and preceptors with preceptorship as an explicit part of their job description and workplace objectives. It is important that the preceptor role is identified as distinct from the mentor role because the NQN requires specific types of support through transition from student to RN rather than continued formal education and educational assessment to meet professional requirements. The difference between student and NQN learning needs is that an appropriate relationship of the more experienced RN supporting the less experienced RN takes place instead of the continuation of the assessment role as undertaken by a student's mentor.

The supernumerary time tool

The research findings strongly support a period of time when NQNs are counted as supernumerary to the established numbers on the ward, department or team. This provides time for the NQN to begin their transition into their new role and develop their role with confidence while being supported.

The supernumerary time tool is intended to predict the length of supernumerary time likely to be needed based on the NQN's experience immediately prior to qualifying. It provides evidence-based guidance to predict the individual needs of NQNs based on the findings of the research. This should be approached with caution and needs to be used in combination with discussion between the NQN and

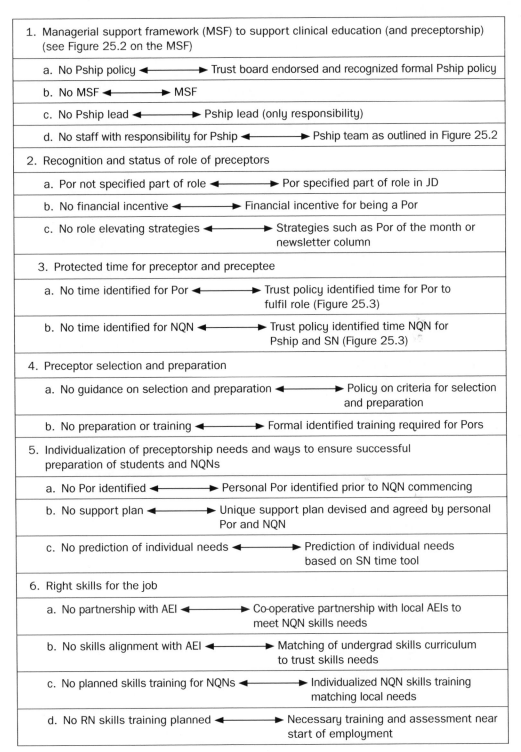

1. Managerial support framework (MSF) to support clinical education (and preceptorship) (see Figure 25.2 on the MSF)

   a. No Pship policy ←——————→ Trust board endorsed and recognized formal Pship policy

   b. No MSF ←————→ MSF

   c. No Pship lead ←——————→ Pship lead (only responsibility)

   d. No staff with responsibility for Pship ←——————→ Pship team as outlined in Figure 25.2

2. Recognition and status of role of preceptors

   a. Por not specified part of role ←——————→ Por specified part of role in JD

   b. No financial incentive ←——————→ Financial incentive for being a Por

   c. No role elevating strategies ←——————→ Strategies such as Por of the month or newsletter column

3. Protected time for preceptor and preceptee

   a. No time identified for Por ←——————→ Trust policy identified time for Por to fulfil role (Figure 25.3)

   b. No time identified for NQN ←——————→ Trust policy identified time NQN for Pship and SN (Figure 25.3)

4. Preceptor selection and preparation

   a. No guidance on selection and preparation ←——————→ Policy on criteria for selection and preparation

   b. No preparation or training ←——————→ Formal identified training required for Pors

5. Individualization of preceptorship needs and ways to ensure successful preparation of students and NQNs

   a. No Por identified ←——————→ Personal Por identified prior to NQN commencing

   b. No support plan ←——————→ Unique support plan devised and agreed by personal Por and NQN

   c. No prediction of individual needs ←——————→ Prediction of individual needs based on SN time tool

6. Right skills for the job

   a. No partnership with AEI ←——————→ Co-operative partnership with local AEIs to meet NQN skills needs

   b. No skills alignment with AEI ←——————→ Matching of undergrad skills curriculum to trust skills needs

   c. No planned skills training for NQNs ←——————→ Individualized NQN skills training matching local needs

   d. No RN skills training planned ←——————→ Necessary training and assessment near start of employment

Figure 25.1 Organizational support tool [Move slider to the *right* to improve preceptorship]

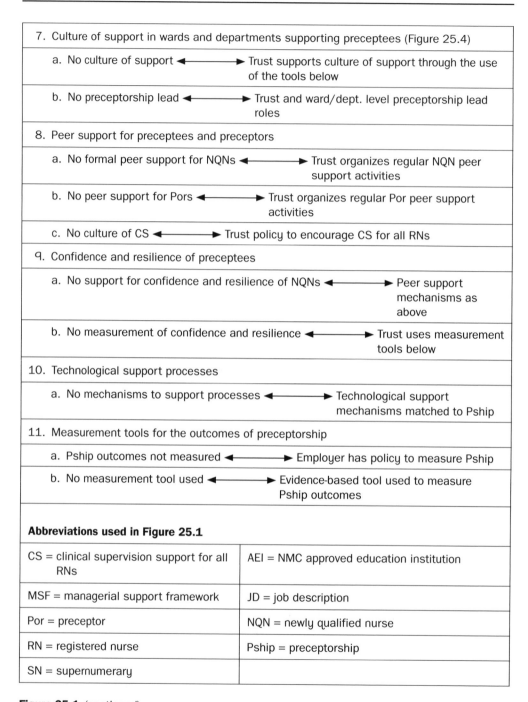

7. Culture of support in wards and departments supporting preceptees (Figure 25.4)

    a. No culture of support ⟷ Trust supports culture of support through the use of the tools below

    b. No preceptorship lead ⟷ Trust and ward/dept. level preceptorship lead roles

8. Peer support for preceptees and preceptors

    a. No formal peer support for NQNs ⟷ Trust organizes regular NQN peer support activities

    b. No peer support for Pors ⟷ Trust organizes regular Por peer support activities

    c. No culture of CS ⟷ Trust policy to encourage CS for all RNs

9. Confidence and resilience of preceptees

    a. No support for confidence and resilience of NQNs ⟷ Peer support mechanisms as above

    b. No measurement of confidence and resilience ⟷ Trust uses measurement tools below

10. Technological support processes

    a. No mechanisms to support processes ⟷ Technological support mechanisms matched to Pship

11. Measurement tools for the outcomes of preceptorship

    a. Pship outcomes not measured ⟷ Employer has policy to measure Pship

    b. No measurement tool used ⟷ Evidence-based tool used to measure Pship outcomes

Abbreviations used in Figure 25.1

CS = clinical supervision support for all RNs	AEI = NMC approved education institution
MSF = managerial support framework	JD = job description
Por = preceptor	NQN = newly qualified nurse
RN = registered nurse	Pship = preceptorship
SN = supernumerary	

Figure 25.1 (*continued*)

Preceptorship lead (PL)	Full-time managerial and strategic role supporting a team of educators
Ward-based preceptorship support facilitator (PSF)	Usually a part-time role but importantly with a separate job description if the nurse is also undertaking a clinical role. The role is supported and ensured by line management from the PL
Preceptors (of NQNs)	The education role or roles are part of the clinical role of the nurse. These parts of their roles are supported and ensured by the PSF

Figure 25.2 Managerial support framework

Individual NQN experience	Specific ward or department	Rotation
A local university with final placement on this clinical area or similar	2 weeks	2 weeks for each new area
Other university-based student with final placement on a similar clinical area	3 weeks	3 weeks for first ward or department then 2 weeks for each new area
A local university-based student with final placement on a community or other dissimilar placement	3 weeks	3 weeks for first ward or department then 2 weeks for each new area
Other university-based student with final placement on a community or other dissimilar placement	4 weeks	4 weeks for first ward or department then 2 weeks for each new area

Figure 25.3 Supernumerary time tool

Before each NQN starts work, tick off each of the following	✓
Make sure that you have enough preceptors to support NQNs when they arrive	
Ensure that your preceptors have completed the trust-approved preceptor preparation course	
Identify a preceptor prior to the NQN starting work	
Inform all staff that the new worker is an NQN and that they are 'learning the ropes'	
Explain to the ward team that NQNs respond best to a local 'culture of support' rather than just leaving their integration into the ward/department to their named preceptor	
Encourage staff to be tolerant of NQNs' inexperience and advise them that if properly encouraged the NQN will become a useful and efficient colleague more quickly	
Encourage the ward/department team to integrate the NQN into their work routine by helping them to learn the specific needs of patients and multidisciplinary team (MDT) in their area	
At regular intervals or more often if necessary, tick off each of the following: 1. Monitor their personal preceptorship progress towards independent RN through reports from their personal preceptor. 2. Monitor the NQN's integration into the ward/dept.	✓
2 weeks after starting work	
1 month after starting work	
3 months after starting work	
6 months after starting work	
If any of the above are unsatisfactory, discuss with the Trust preceptorship lead and create an action plan to remedy the situation	
When preceptorship is agreed to be completed by the ward/department preceptorship lead, the preceptor and the NQN inform the Trust preceptorship lead for their records	

Figure 25.4 Local culture of support tool

preceptor, as each NQN will have their individual needs assessed and supported by their preceptor and the workforce community (Figure 25.4). For example, the research findings supported the hypothesis that NQNs who had their final placement in the ward or department where they commenced their first post would need less time to 'settle in'. Those who had completed their pre-registration programme with placements in the same hospital but not on the specific ward or department may need longer and those who had never had placements at the trust would probably require the most support. Nevertheless, as stated earlier, this is not universally the case but it is worth while to consider when supporting NQNs as individuals.

The local culture of support tool

In this research it was found that the 'culture of support' on some wards and departments was in many ways more important than the overall organizational preceptorship framework or even the individual one-to-one preceptorship support provided by the named preceptor for the NQN. This support tool is intended to provide wards and departments with evidence-based advice on the best methods to support NQNs.

The matron or sister should identify a preceptorship lead for each ward/department. This will usually be the ward-based preceptorship support facilitator (PSF) but can be any named individual. A record of these preceptorship leads should be kept by the Trust preceptorship lead.

The ward/department preceptorship lead to complete this checklist for each NQN entering the ward/department (Figure 25.4).

NQNs identified that they were better supported if their ward or department had a 'preceptorship culture' or 'culture of support' as described in Figure 25.4. This was identified by NQNs as being in need of additional support for a period of time with responsibility of a team to support transition. This was because their named preceptor could not always work on the same shift as them and the realities of practice meant that it was possible they would be working in a different team or with other patients in a different part of the ward. The opposite of this 'culture of support' is what Halpin (2015) has described in her recent research as 'incivility' that leads to one of the most destructive stressors for the NQN. Kelly and Ahern (2009) went further and described this behaviour by experienced nurses as 'eating their young'. Clearly, therefore, it would be advantageous to organizations to foster a culture of support at ward and department level to counter the destructive attitudes encapsulated in the culture of incivility described in Halpin's (2015) thesis and to encourage the supportive aspects described by the participants in this study as a culture of support (Whitehead *et al.*, 2016).

If the four parts of this toolkit, presented in Figures 25.1–25.4, are implemented by an employer they will provide the most up-to-date, evidence-based support to facilitate an environment that will aid recruitment, retention and skills development in NQNs. From the perspective of the NQN, it will reduce the stress of the process and speed the acquisition of skills and knowledge required to be an experienced and respected member of the RN team.

Reflection

- Consider the toolkit described above with a view to how the implementation of this could help your transition.
- How can you use the toolkit to understand and aid your own transition?

Method of measuring your experience of transition from student to RN

The main aspects of the transition process have been outlined above. A framework has been suggested for measuring your own progress through the clinical skills development, knowledge acquisition and emotional journey identified by the research and this is shown in Figure 25.5.

List the skills you will need to develop below	Date when you feel that you have mastered these
e.g. medications management and administration	
List the medical conditions common to your patients in your workplace below	Date when you feel that you have studied sufficiently to understand these at the necessary level
e.g. chronic obstructive pulmonary disease (COPD)	
List the multidisciplinary team (MDT) roles necessary to care for your patients below	Date when you feel that you have studied sufficiently to understand these at the necessary level
e.g. role of the social worker	
List the administrative duties and information technology (IT)-related activities necessary to care for your patients below	Date when you feel that you have studied sufficiently to understand these at the necessary level
e.g. how to request blood results	
Refer to the strengths, weaknesses, opportunities and threats (SWOT) analysis completed in Chapter 23 and make a list of actions to achieve your objectives below	Date when you feel that you have completed each action generated from the SWOT
e.g. improving self-confidence in your ability to practise the skills important for patient care in your workplace	

Figure 25.5 Method of measuring your experience of transition

Conclusion

This chapter has provided an insight into the things considered by good employers when constructing support for NQNs. Reflection on this should help you to provide a framework to help you to make your own journey from student to RN as well as selecting the best employer to work for.

References

Halpin, Y. (2015) *Newly Qualified Nurse Transition: Stress Experiences and Stress-mediating Factors – a Longitudinal Study.* PhD thesis. London Southbank University.

Kelly, J. and Ahern, K. (2009) Preparing nurses for practice: a phenomenological study of the new graduate in Australia, *Journal of Clinical Nursing*, 18(6): 910–918.

Whitehead, B., Owen, P., Holmes, D., Beddingham, E., Simmons, M., Henshaw, L., Barton, M. and Walker, C. (2013) Supporting newly qualified nurses in the UK: a systematic literature review, *Nurse Education Today*, 33(4): 370–377.

Whitehead, B., Owen, P., Henshaw, L., Beddingham, E. and Simmons, M. (2016) Supporting newly qualified nurse transition: a case study in a UK hospital, *Nurse Education Today*, 36: 58–63.

Index

abstracts, reading 18, 20
abuse 119–20
  forms of 119
academic content 5–6
academic credibility 39
academic writing *see* writing
accountability 90, 91–2
Adair, J. 27
adjourning 114–15
affective domain 31–2
agency posts 107
Ahern, K. 155
Allan, H.T. 102, 129
applications for a job 50, 51,
  105–10
assessment 130, 135
  of academic writing 39–43
  final year of course 3, 7–8,
    35–6, 37–44
  of patients *see* patient
    assessment
  rationale for 39–41
  sign-off mentor assessment
    50, 51, 101–4
assignment writing 10–12
  example plan 11–12
attitudes 31–2
autocratic leadership 24–5
autonomy 122

Bach, S. 25, 91, 130
BBC *Panorama* programme
  120–1
Beauchamp, T.L. 122
Belbin, M.R. 26, 28
beneficence 122
Benne, K.D. 114, 117
Benner, P.E. 32, 56, 114
Bennis, W.G. 26, 79
Berne, E. 62
Biggs, J. 32
Bloom's taxonomy 31–2
British Nursing Index (BNI) 19

Brock, M. 145, 146, 147
Brown, M. 145, 146, 147
burnout 145

Care Act 2014 121
careers advisers 107
carers, teaching 30
caseload management in a
  primary care setting 50,
  86–9
challenges 39–40
Childress, J.F. 122
clinical competency
  continuum 32, 55–6, 114
Clinical Nurse Educator
  Network 135
clinical supervision 130–1
clinical technology skills
  96, 97
coaching 91, 130
Cochrane Library of
  systematic reviews 19
Code of the NMC 28, 30, 54,
  90, 101, 121
cognitive domain 31–2
communication 7
  importance in patient
    assessment 70–1
  learning from communica-
    tion with patients 76
  in sign-off mentor assess-
    ment 102–4
  skills 60, 62–4, 68, 96
community nursing 50, 86–9
compassion 57, 71, 104, 144–5
competence
  clinical competency
    continuum 32, 55–6, 114
  demonstrating in the
    sign-off mentor assess-
    ment 50, 51, 101–4
  practising as a staff nurse
    64–5

thinking like a staff nurse
  56–9
conclusion 12, 18, 20
confidence 125, 139–43
  building up 140–2
  in your abilities 47–50
  practising as a staff nurse
    64–5
  temporary loss of 55–6,
    139–40
consent 76–7
core values 57–8
criticality 11, 12–13
criticism of NQNs 115–17
crossed transaction
  communications 63–4
Cullum, N. 16
culture of support 125, 126,
  136–7, 140, 149, 150,
  154, 155
Cumulative Index to Nursing
  and Allied Health
  Literature (CINAHL) 19

database searches 18–20
Deane, M. 14, 39
decision making 79–83
  sign-off mentor assessment
    102–3
delegation 38–9
  assisting staff you have
    delegated to 99
  demonstrating in sign-off
    mentor assessment 102–3
  leadership and 23, 28, 92–4
  staff nurse skills 50, 51, 83,
    90–4, 97, 98–9
deontology 79, 121–2
  management 80–1
Department of Health (DH)
  67, 119
  preceptorship 129, 134, 135
descriptive text 12–13, 41

dignity 57
directing 91
discharge from hospital 87–8
domains of learning 31–2
Drennan, J. 60
dress 109
drug administration 38, 88, 100, 116
Duchscher, J.E. 129, 140
dysfunctional roles 117

educational taxonomies 31–2
Ellis, P. 25, 91, 130
Emmers-Sommer, T.M. 70
emotional distress 68–70
empathy 57
    impact of not showing 68–70
enablers 39–40
engagement 4
Essential Skills Clusters 95–6, 140
ethics 79–83
    leadership 81–3
    management 80–1
    regarding raising concerns 121–2
evidence
    on becoming an NQN 124–8
    hierarchies of 13, 17–18
evidence-based practice (EBP) 16–22, 77–8, 104, 118, 124
    importance in final student year 21
    importance in first year as an NQN 21–2
    systematic reviews 17–21
expectations of staff nurses 56–7, 73–5
expert role 55–6
extrinsic motivation 39–40

facilitation of one-to-one preceptorship 125, 126, 149, 150–4
feedback 109–10
final year course 3–8
    academic content 5–6
    practice content 6–7
Fineout-Overholt, E. 16

fitness to join the register 47–53
forming 114–15
four principles approach to biomedical ethics 121–2
functional roles of group members 114, 117
fundamental care 65, 97, 98

Gauthier, T. 145–6
general care 65, 97, 98
Gill, G. 28
Goleman, D. 27
Gopee, N. 14, 39
groups
    dynamics of 4–5
    functional roles of members 114, 117
    stages of small group development 114–15
    see also teamworking

Halpin, Y. 126, 155
Havn, V. 13
Haywood, M. 120–1
Healthcare Leadership Model 93–4
hierarchies of evidence 13, 17–18
holistic care 50, 67–72, 95, 97
hospital ward team leadership 50, 79–85
hub and spoke model for placements 48
Hyde, A. 60

incivility 115–17, 126, 155
individualistic roles 117
individualized preceptorship programmes 125, 126, 149, 150–4
information technology (IT) skills 97
internet search engines 19
interviews, job 108–9
intrinsic motivation 39–40

Jensen, M. 114–15
Joanna Briggs Institute library of systematic reviews 19

job advertisements 107
job applications 50, 51, 105–10
job changes 136
job fairs 106
job searches 106–7
justice 122

Keeling, J. 3–4, 57
Kelly, J. 155
key skills for a staff nurse 50, 51, 95–100
keywords 18, 19
knowing your limitations 47–50, 109, 142
knowledge 31–2
    of your speciality 50, 73–8, 103
    practising as a staff nurse 60–2
knowledgeable doer 58, 60
Kramer, M. 125, 129, 140

laissez-faire leadership 92–3
leadership 23–9, 42
    delegation and 23, 28, 92–4
    demonstrating in the sign-off mentor assessment 102–3
    ethical 81–3
    of a hospital ward team 50, 79–85
    linking theory and practice 27–8, 79–83
    vs management 26–7, 79–80
    primary care settings 50, 86–9
learning
    domains of 31–2
    methods 75–7
    reflective 36, 54, 76–7, 77–8
    resources for 74–5
    responsibility for your own learning 73–5, 77
    taking advantage of all learning experiences 137
learning curve 38
learning outcomes 41
legislation
    on raising concerns 121
    see also under individual Acts

limitations
    knowing your own
        limitations 47–50,
        109, 142
    on searches 18, 19–20
literature review 11
local culture of support 125,
    126, 136–7, 140, 149, 150,
    154, 155
logical progression 43
lying 80, 82

Maben, J. 115
Malnutrition Universal
    Screening Tool 71
management 23–9
    ethical 80–1
    hospital ward team 50,
        79–85
    leadership vs 26–7,
        79–80
    primary care settings 50,
        86–9
managerial support
    framework 125, 126, 149,
        150, 153
Manning, J. 97
marking criteria 41
Martin, V. 93
measuring progress in
    transition 155–6
media 120–1
medication administration 38,
    88, 100, 116
meetings with the preceptor
    137
Melnyk, B. 16
Mental Capacity Act 2005 77,
    120, 121
mentoring 42, 91, 130, 135
    sign-off mentor assessment
        50, 51, 101–4
Menzies, I.E.P. 139
mind mapping 42, 43
mindfulness 144, 145–7
    programmes 145–6
miscommunication 62–4
Modified Early Warning
    System 71
multidisciplinary team (MDT)
    84–5, 87–8

National Patient Safety
    Agency (NPSA) *Five
    Steps to Safer Surgery* 81
Neff, K.D. 146
networks of support 125, 126,
    140
Nilsson, K. 140
non-maleficence 122
norming 114–15
novice–expert progression
    32, 55–6, 114
nursing degree programme
    9–10, 58, 139
Nursing and Midwifery
    Council (NMC) 5, 30
    Code 28, 30, 54, 90, 101, 121
    Essential Skills Clusters
        95–6, 140
    Margaret Haywood 120–1
    pin number 107
    preceptorship 134–5
    raising concerns 51–2, 118,
        119, 120, 121, 130
    revalidation 76
    *Standards to Support
    Learning and
    Assessment in
    Practice* 30

observation skills 96
Odland, L. 13
organizational support 125,
    126, 149, 150, 151–2
orientation 38

Panorama programme
    120–1
patient assessment 67–72
    tools for 71
patient-centred approach
    67–9
patient empowerment 67–8
patient group direction
    (PGD) 88, 100
patient specific directions 88,
    100
patients 55
    learning from
        communication with 76
    leaving patients in a
        distressed state 68–70

perceptions of staff nurses
    56–7
    teaching 30
Pederson, S.N. 70
peer review 14
peer support 14, 125
    groups 131, 137
performing 114–15
personal roles 117
personal statement 107–8
Phillips, C. 106
PICO 19
plagiarism 14
planning
    academic writing 42, 43
    teaching plans 33–4, 35
practice
    content of the final year
        course 6–7
    linking theory and 6, 13,
        27–8, 35, 43, 79–83
    practising as a staff nurse
        50, 60–6
    using evidence on precep-
        torship to improve 126–7
preceptorship 54, 109, 129,
    134–8
    ensuring a good experience
        137
    finding out about 135–7
    meeting with the preceptor
        129–30
    research evidence on
        124–8
    support toolkit 126, 149–57
preceptorship support
    facilitator (PSF) 155
Preferred Reporting Items for
    Systematic Reviews and
    Meta-Analyses
    (PRISMA) 18
preparation
    for job interviews 108
    for placement 75
prescribing 97
primary care settings 50,
    86–9
professionalism 3–5, 57,
    103–4
progress measurement
    155–6

Project 2000 nursing
    programme 9, 58
psychomotor domain 31–2
Public Concern at Work 121
Public Interest Disclosure Act
    1998 121

questions
  assignment writing
    question 10–11
  job interviews 109

raising concerns 51–2, 118–23
reality shock 125, 140
  dealing with 129–33
reasoning, communicating
  102–3
recommendations 12, 18,
  20–1, 43
referencing 10, 13
referrals 10
reflection 36, 54, 76–7, 77–8
reflective assignments
  10–11
registration, fitness for
  47–53
reliability 4
reports 10–11
research
  evidence-based practice
    16–22, 77–8, 104, 124
  evidence on becoming and
    NQN 124–8
  on prospective employers
    108
  on your speciality 76–7, 103
  systematic reviews 17–21,
    124–7
resilience 116, 126, 144–8
  interventions 145–6
resources for learning 74–5
revalidation 76
Rieber, L.J. 14
Ritchie, D. 5
roles
  functional group roles 114,
    117
  team roles 26
Royal College of Nursing 144
rules 80–1, 83
  breaking bad rules 82

Scarf, V. 145
searches
  of databases 18–20
  job 106–7
self-awareness 144–5
self-compassion 144–5,
  146–7
self-questioning 55–6
Sheats, P. 114, 117
Sherratt, L. 48
sign-off mentor assessment
  50, 51, 101–4
skills 31–2, 139–40
  acquiring after qualifying
    127
  confidence in and fitness to
    join the register 47–50
  for hospital ward patient
    group management 83–4
  key skills for the staff
    nurse 50, 51, 95–100
  practising as a staff nurse
    60–2
social roles 117
speaking out 51–2, 118–23
speciality
  knowledge of 50, 73–8, 103
  researching 76–7, 103
speed of working 116–17
SPICE 19
stages of small group
  development 114–15
Standing, M. 13
storming 114–15
strengths, limitations,
  opportunities and
  challenges (SLOC)
  analysis 49, 58–9
strengths, weaknesses,
  opportunities and threats
  (SWOT) analysis 141–2
stress-reduction interventions
  145–6
Structure of the Observed
  Learning Outcome
  (SOLO) taxonomy 32
structure of written work
  11–12, 41–3
supernumary time 125, 126,
  149, 150–4
supervision, clinical 130–1

support
  dealing with reality shock
    129–33
  for learning 75
  local culture of 125, 126,
    136–7, 140, 149, 150, 154,
    155
  managerial support
    framework 125, 126, 149,
    150, 153
  networks 125, 126, 140
  organizational 125, 126,
    149, 150, 151–2
  peer support 14, 125, 131,
    137
  preceptorship *see*
    preceptorship
surgery, safety in 81
systematic reviews 17–21
  research on preceptorship
    124–5, 126

table of articles 18, 20
Tang, C. 32
task roles 117
taxonomies, educational
  31–2
teaching 30–6
teaching cycle 33, 35
teaching plans 33–4, 35
team roles 26
teamworking 4–5, 25–6, 28,
  42, 51–2
  assessing abilities in 39
  becoming a team player
    113–17
  criticism from other team
    members 115–17
  multidisciplinary team
    (MDT) 84–5, 87–8
technology skills 96, 97
Templeman, J. 3–4, 57
theory–practice links 6, 13,
  27–8, 35, 43, 79–83
thinking like a staff nurse 50,
  54–9
Thomas, J. 130
titles 18, 20
toolkit for transition 126,
  149–57
transactional analysis 62–4

transformational
    leadership 93
transition shock *see* reality
    shock
Trust clearing activities 107
truth telling 80, 82
Tuckman, B. 114–15

UK Clinical Nurse Educator
    Network 135
uncertainty 55–6
United Kingdom Central
    Council for Nursing
    Midwifery and Health
    Visiting (UKCC) 9, 58, 129
utilitarianism 79, 121–2
    leadership 81–3

value
    becoming a valuable team
        member 113–17
    demonstrating one's value
        at an early stage 113–15
    valuing colleagues/staff
        92, 93
values 5
    core 57–8
Vedi, C. 13
vocation, sense of 57

ward team leadership 50,
    79–85
Webb, L. 10
Whistleblower Interview
    Project 121

whistleblowing 120–1
Whitehead, B. 113, 124–5, 126,
    129, 140, 149
Whitehead, D. 41
World Health Organization
    (WHO) 70
    *Surgical Safety
        Checklist
        Guidance* 81
writing 5–6, 9–15
    assessment of 39–43
    assignments 10–12
    criticality 11, 12–13
    structuring 11–12, 41–3
Wynd, C.A. 57

Yoder-Wise, P.S. 25